HOSPITAL WASTE MANAGEMENT
A Guide for Self Assessment and Review

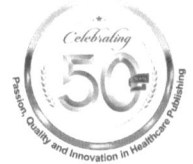

HOSPITAL WASTE MANAGEMENT
A Guide for Self Assessment and Review

SECOND EDITION

Shishir Basarkar MBBS, PGDHHM, MBA, Dip T&D
Chief Operating Officer
Bansal Superspeciality Hospital
Bhopal, Madhya Pradesh, India

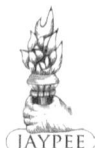

JAYPEE BROTHERS MEDICAL PUBLISHERS
The Health Sciences Publisher
New Delhi | London

Jaypee Brothers Medical Publishers (P) Ltd

Headquarter

Jaypee Brothers Medical Publishers (P) Ltd
EMCA House, 23/23-B
Ansari Road, Daryaganj
New Delhi 110 002, India
Landline: +91-11-23272143, +91-11-23272703
+91-11-23282021, +91-11-23245672
Email: jaypee@jaypeebrothers.com

Corporate Office

Jaypee Brothers Medical Publishers (P) Ltd
4838/24, Ansari Road, Daryaganj
New Delhi 110 002, India
Phone: +91-11-43574357
Fax: +91-11-43574314
Email: jaypee@jaypeebrothers.com
Website: www.jaypeebrothers.com
Website: www.jaypeedigital.com

Overseas Office

J.P. Medical Ltd
83 Victoria Street, London
SW1H 0HW (UK)
Phone: +44 20 3170 8910
Fax: +44 (0)20 3008 6180
Email: info@jpmedpub.com

© 2021, Jaypee Brothers Medical Publishers

The views and opinions expressed in this book are solely those of the original contributor(s)/author(s) and do not necessarily represent those of editor(s) of the book.

All rights reserved. No part of this publication may be reproduced, stored or transmitted in any form or by any means, electronic, mechanical, photocopying, recording or otherwise, without the prior permission in writing of the publishers.

All brand names and product names used in this book are trade names, service marks, trademarks or registered trademarks of their respective owners. The publisher is not associated with any product or vendor mentioned in this book.

Medical knowledge and practice change constantly. This book is designed to provide accurate, authoritative information about the subject matter in question. However, readers are advised to check the most current information available on procedures included and check information from the manufacturer of each product to be administered, to verify the recommended dose, formula, method and duration of administration, adverse effects and contraindications. It is the responsibility of the practitioner to take all appropriate safety precautions. Neither the publisher nor the author(s)/editor(s) assume any liability for any injury and/or damage to persons or property arising from or related to use of material in this book.

This book is sold on the understanding that the publisher is not engaged in providing professional medical services. If such advice or services are required, the services of a competent medical professional should be sought.

Every effort has been made where necessary to contact holders of copyright to obtain permission to reproduce copyright material. If any have been inadvertently overlooked, the publisher will be pleased to make the necessary arrangements at the first opportunity. The **CD/DVD-ROM** (if any) provided in the sealed envelope with this book is complimentary and free of cost. **Not meant for sale.**

Inquiries for bulk sales may be solicited at: jaypee@jaypeebrothers.com

Hospital Waste Management: A Guide for Self Assessment and Review

First Edition: 2009

Second Edition: **2021**

ISBN: 978-93-88958-51-6

Printed at Repro India Limited

Dedicated to

*My Family Members
and
Teachers*

PREFACE TO THE SECOND EDITION

I am singularly previleged to bring out second edition of the book *"Hospital Waste Management: A Guide for Self Assessment and Review"* in collaboration with M/s Jaypee Brothers Medical Publishers.

Though I tried my level best to make the content simple, yet comprehensive to understand the basic of Biomedical Waste Management. However if you find any inadequacy, then please write to me on my e-mail: shishirbasarkar@yahoo.co.in.

I would be deeply indebted for direct or indirect support to bring out improvement.

Happy Reading!

Shishir Basarkar

PREFACE TO THE FIRST EDITION

This book is a humble attempt to familiarize all medical and paramedical professionals with the importance of hospital waste management. The purpose of the book will be well served if the finer points are inculcated and brought into attitude. Indeed, the objective of this book is not to make the specialist but rather to serve as an appetizer for further reading on the subject.

Our own wrong habits make authorities to bring out various laws and rules which then force us to abide by them, hence the book attempts to emphasize and enhance the competency of the professionals by having proper knowledge about hospital waste and hazards associated with it.

Any waste, whatever it may be, should not be handled indiscriminately because it may lead patients as well as healthcare workers to catastrophic situation culminating to fatal infections. The situation further gets more difficult if negligence is done in treatment, reporting and preventing further occurrence.

I have tried to simplify the subject by presenting each topic in short answers form so that each question is well understood. I also tried to give line diagrams of complex processes and machines, thus making them easy to understand. However, it does not resist the reader to the classical reading scheme as one does not necessarily have to begin from first page and run through to the end. Attempts have been made to make every chapter complete in itself, therefore, it is possible to pick out single chapter without losing the track.

Shishir Basarkar

ACKNOWLEDGMENTS

I wish to express my sincere thanks and indebtedness to my entire teachers for their valuable teaching which made me capable to conceptualize and bring out this book.

I like to thank my family members who every time supported me.

I also express my deepest thanks to Dr Chandrahas Kulkarni who showed undoubted faith in my capabilities and this book is the result of that faith.

My sincere acknowledgment to Dr Shivani Tandon who tirelessly worked for editing the manuscript to bring out in present form.

My wife Dr Rashmi and daughters Nimisha and Samiksha deserve special complements for giving me moral support, encouragement and required space while working on second edition. All of them supported me unconditionally throughout my working on this book.

Last, but not the least I would like to thank M/s Jaypee Brothers Medical Publishers (P) Ltd, New Delhi, for publishing and printing of this book.

CONTENTS

Abbreviations	*xv*
Introduction	*xvii*
1. Our Environment	1
2. Hospital Waste	5
3. Effect of Hospital Waste on Environment and Health	18
4. Generation and Segregation	32
5. Transport and Storage	44
6. Treatment and Disposal of Waste	53
7. Education and Training	79
8. Managerial Issues in Biomedical Waste Management	93
9. New Concept in Biomedical Waste Management	113
10. Laws Related to Biomedical Waste Management	116
11. Infection Control	138
12. Occupational Hazards and Universal Precaution	146
13. Mercury Waste Management	157
14. Management of Specialized Waste	172
15. Cytotoxic Waste Management	179
16. Disinfectants in Hospital	187
17. Biomedical Waste Management in COVID-19	197
Key Concepts	*203*
Annexures	*217*
Further Readings	*259*

ABBREVIATIONS

AD	:	Automatic Disabled
AERB	:	Atomic Energy Regulatory Board
AIDS	:	Acquired Immuno Dificiency Syndrome
ANM	:	Auxillary Nurse Midwife
APC	:	Anti Pollution Control
APCD	:	Air Pollution Control Device
AYUSH	:	Ayurveda, Yoga, Unani, Siddha, Homeopathy
BARC	:	Bhabha Atomic Research Center
BMWM	:	Biomedical Waste Management
BOD	:	Biological Oxygen Demand
BP	:	Blood Pressure
CAPA	:	Corrective Action and Preventive Action
CBWTF	:	Common Biomedical Waste Treatment Facility
CE	:	Combustion Efficiency
CHC	:	Community Health Center
CNS	:	Central Nervous System
COD	:	Chemical Oxygen Demand
CPCB	:	Central Pollution Control Board
CSSD	:	Central Sterile Supply Department
DEHP	:	Diethylhexyl Phthalate
DMO	:	District Medical Officer
EC	:	Exposure Code
ERP	:	Extended Producer's Responsibility
ETP	:	Effluent Treatment Plant
GSCM	:	Green Supply Chain Management
HBV	:	Hepatitis B Virus
HCV	:	Hepatitis C Virus
HCW	:	Health Care Worker
HIV	:	Human Immunodeficiency Virus
HW	:	Hazardous Waste
ICN	:	Infection Control Nurse
ICO	:	Infection Control Officer
ICT	:	Infection Control Team
ICU	:	Intensive Care Unit
ISO	:	International Standard Organization

KSA	:	Knowledge, Skill, Attitude
MO	:	Medical Officer
MPW	:	Multi Purpose Worker
OPD	:	Out Patient Department
OT	:	Operation Theater
PATH	:	Programme for Appropriate Technology in Health
PDCA	:	Plan, Do, Check, Act
PHC	:	Primary Health Center
PIL	:	Public Interest Litigation
PLC	:	Programmable Logic Control
PPE	:	Personal Protective Equipment
PPM	:	Parts Per Million
PSI	:	Pounds Per Square Inch
PVC	:	Poly Vinyl Chloride
RNTCP	:	Revised National Tuberculosis Control Programme
RPM	:	Revolutions Per Minute
SC	:	Status Code
SOP	:	Standing Order Procedure
SPCB	:	State Pollution Control Board
STP	:	Sewage Treatment Plant
TNI	:	Training Need Identification
TSDF	:	Treatement, Storage, Disposal facility
WC	:	Water Column

INTRODUCTION

The serious concern of the healthcare facilities is the generation of biomedical waste, which is hazardous to health of community and people who are associated with handling of the waste. Various national and international environmental and health agencies have shown their concern towards these wastes as they may cause serious infectious diseases like hepatitis, tuberculosis and HIV/AIDS. Most of the hospitals do not have effective disposal system leading to complex problem of hygiene and sanitation in hospitals.

Hospital generated waste is disposed off illegally into the Municipal garbage and drainage system.

In developing countries, very often the Municipal workers get pricking injuries from needles, sharps and broken glass pieces. The other infectious waste which creates complex environmental problem is radioactive waste which has prolonged half-life and needs very sophisticated and appropriate system for ultimate disposal.

Though the use of disposal items have reduced the rate of infection but at the same time has increased the volume of the waste which needs to be disposed properly.

Because of the concerns shown by national and international agencies the notification of the Biomedical Waste (Management and Handling) Rules, 1998 was brought out by Union Ministry of Environment and Forests under the provision of Environment (Protection) Act, 1986. Under these rules, all healthcare institutions are found to make necessary arrangements for proper handling and management of waste, failing of which, the head of the institution is liable for punishment.

Effective waste disposal can be achieved only by considering the various components of the waste management system and this should be made integral part of the hospital planning and designing of the hospital.

Chapter 1

Our Environment

1. **What is the definition of Environment?**
   It is the constant interaction between living beings and various surrounding factors like physical (water, soil, heat), social (habits, customs, occupation) and biological (human, plants, animal).

2. **What is biosphere and what are its main subdivision?**
   Biosphere is the part of earth where people live and it has 3 subdivision namely lithosphere (solid), hydrosphere (liquid) and atmosphere (gas).

3. **What is 10% law?**
   At every level of trophic level 10% of energy is transferred to next level of the previous level, and this is due to energy loss at every level because of:
   - Part of energy utilized by organism for its body activities.
   - Part of energy is not available to organism itself.
   - Some organisms one not consumed by next trophic level so undergo decomposition.

4. **What do you understand by ecosystem?**
   It is a self-sustaining and self-regulating system which is the result of the interaction of an individual organisms with each other and at the same time with physical components of environment too.

5. **What is top soil?**
   It is the fertile soil which covers the few inches of the earth surface and is rich in organic matter.

6. **What are essential components of ecosystem?**
   Two components are of ecosystem:

1. ***Abiotic:*** These are non-living like light, soil, air, water, etc.
2. ***Biotic:*** These are living components like plant, animals, human and microbes.

Biotic components is dependent on abiotic component for survival.

7. **What do you understand by biomagnification?**

   When there is gradual increase in the concentration of chemicals as they pass through higher levels in the food chain is known as biomagnification. It is also called bioaccumulation.

8. **Few words about trophic level.**

   Organism belongs to certain class as per their source of food supply and this class is called trophic level.

   The word trophic (Gr) means nourishment

9. **How many trophic levels are there?**

   There are 3 trophic levels:

Ist level	Producer	Plants	Grass
II level	Primary consumer	Grazers	Dear
III level	Secondary consumer	Predator	Tiger

10. **What is the difference between food chain and food web?**

    Food chain: When the food energy is transferred through the chain of organisms from one trophic level to another.

    Food web: Network of the food chains at different trophic level and at one level the source may be different (Fig. 1.1).

11. **Write few words about different types of food chain?**
    - Predator – prey food drain – Butterfly
    - Detritus (decomposed organic matter) food chain – vultures
    - Parasitic food chain – worms in bowel.

12. **What is the impact of biomedical waste on human and environmental health?**

Type of waste	Impact
Anatomical waste	Infections get transmitted through either direct contact or vectors
Laboratory cultures, specimen, vaccines and live microorganisms	Various health disorders like cough, eye redness and burning, skin burn, skin itching, dermatitis are caused when non-treated waste comes in contact.

    Contd...

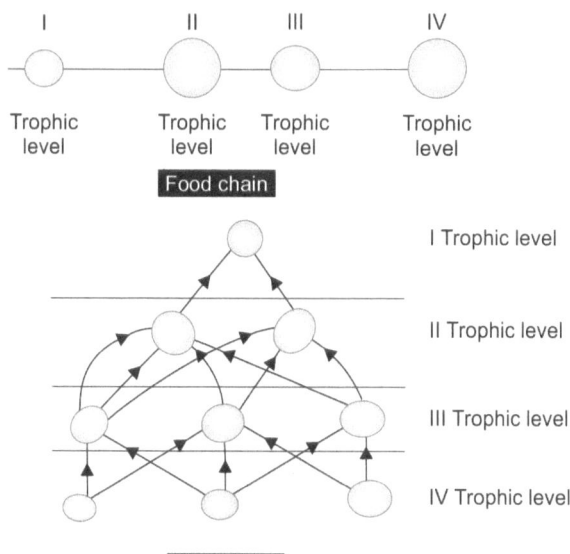

Fig. 1.1: Food chain and food web.

Contd...

Type of waste	Impact
Blood, body fluids, cotton swabs, bandages	Transmission of infections like hepatitis, tuberculosis, enteric fever, and AIDS, etc. either through vectors or by direct contacts
Waste sharps (scalpel, needles, broken glasses, blades)	Transmission of infections like tetanus, hepatitis, septicemia, AIDS, etc. by direct innoculations
Catheters and plastic tubing, PVC surgical gloves	Dissolution of DHEP chemical from PVC material may serve as human carcinogens and may disturb hormonal function in person in close contact
IV fluid bottles, blood collection bags and urine-bags	On incineration these products release dioxin and furan, suspended particulate matter, and gases. These articles may get illegally recycled and further aid to spread of infection
Chemical waste (used in disinfections process)	Causes cough, and headache on exposure, on prolong reaction in human body affects normal function of hormones and acts as carcinogens

Contd...

Contd...

Type of waste	Impact
Cytotoxic chemical waste like anticancer drugs, phenyl, strong alkalies and acids, radioactive materials	Cytotoxic effect can be manifested in the form of fetal abnormalities, skin diseases, ulcers, cancer and anemia
Incineration ash	Partially incinerated ash may be source of various infections

13. **What are the environmental problems arises from disposal of untreated biomedical waste?**

   Following are environmental problems which arises from disposal of untreated biomedical waste:
   - Decomposing of waste may generate foul and obnoxious odor in the healthcare facility premises or surrounding area.
   - Waste dumps may attract stray animals and birds that will spread the untreated waste material leading to unhygienic and unaesthetic environment.
   - Waste may clog the drainage system leading to unhygienic surrounding environment and may act as breading grounds from flies and mosquitoes which further spread the disease.
   - The ground water may get contaminated by formation of leachate from untreated decomposing waste.
   - Disastrous ecological effects may be produced by contamination of ground water and land by indiscriminate disposal of pharmaceutical waste.
   - Open burning or uncontrolled incineration of waste can generate dioxin and furan gases which causes air pollution.

Chapter 2

Hospital Waste

1. **What is the multi-layered system of rural health care in India?**
   In India the healthcare system is divided at five levels and these are:
   1. *Subcenter:* This is the most basic unit of healthcare delivery system and most peripheral contact point. It caters for about 3000–5000 populations and these subcenters are staffed with one female multipurpose worker (MPW) and one male multipurpose worker. if female MPW is not available then one auxiliary nurse midwife (ANM) is posted at subcenter. in India there are more than 1,47,069 subcenters.
   2. *Primary health center (PHC):* It is a referral unit for six subcenters. It caters for 20,000 to 30,000 population. Each PHC has 4-6 indoor bed for patient admission. The staff at PHC consists of one medical officer (MO) and 14 paramedics. There are more than 23,391 PHCs.
   3. *Community health center (CHC):* It is a referral unit for four PHCs. It is 30 bedded hospital. The staff at CHC consists of doctors, nurses, paramedical and support staff. At present there are more than 5530 CHC in India.
   4. *Sub district hospital:* They are located at the divisional head quarter of each district head quarter level and has bed strength ranging from 100 to 300. These have all the basic specialties.
   5. *District hospital:* These hospitals are located at district level and has bed strength of above 300 beds.

2. **What is waste?**
   Waste is the discarded material much of which can be recycled or reused depending on the type of waste.

3. **What do you mean by word 'waste'?**

   The word 'waste' refers to useless, unused, unwanted or discarded material. It can also be defined as something which is not put in to proper usage at a given time. The waste generation is the result of 'throw away' cultures prevalent everywhere including healthcare sector.

4. **What is the WHO definition of hospital?**

   A hospital is an integral part of a social and medical organization the function of which is to provide for the population complete health care both curative and preventive and whose outpatient services reach out to the family and its home environment.

   It is also a center for the training of health workers and biosocial research.

5. **Other than hospitals what are other sources of biomedical waste generatiosn?**

   The other sources are:
   - Medical research laboratories
   - Tattoo shops and body piercing shops
   - Acupuncture clinics and other clinics practicing alternative medical therapies
   - Blood banks
   - Pathology laboratories
   - Physiotherapy and podiatrists clinics
   - Veterinary hospital and pet clinics
   - Ambulance and special emergency service centers
   - General practitioner's clinics
   - Pharmaceutical plants and medical shops
   - Hospice centers and residential homes for chronically ill patients.

6. **How the biomedical waste is quantified on per patient bed per day basis?**

   The biomedical waste is quantified by using formula:

   Total quantum of waste generated per day (W) divided by total number of patient beds occupied at a time (B).

   $Q = W/D$

7. **How many types of waste are there?**

   There are various types of waste generated in the health care setting. Types of waste are general waste or non-infectious waste, biomedical waste, contaminated waste, pathological waste, animal waste, pressurized cans, infectious waste, chemical waste, liquid waste, hazardous waste, cytotoxic waste, blood and its products waste, radioactive waste, sharps, etc.

8. **What is the difference between sewage and sullage?**

   Sewage it is the waste water containing solid and liquid excreta having very unpleasant smell. Sullage it is the waste water which does not contain human excreta. Example waste water from kitchen, bathroom, etc.

9. **How the waste can be classified in subcategories?**

   Waste can be classified in to various subcategories by multitude of schemes:
   - Based on physical state—solid, liquid, gaseous.
   - Based on material—glass, paper, etc.
   - Based on physical properties—combustible, compostable, recyclable.
   - Based on origin of waste—domestic, commercial, agricultural, industrial, etc.
   - Based on safety level—hazardous, nonhazardous.

   In India, for regulatory purposes, waste is generally classified into municipal solid waste and hazardous waste.

10. **What is an average percentage distribution of waste in hospital?**

    80%—General waste
    15%—Infectious waste
    01%—Sharp waste
    3%—Chemical and pharmacological waste.
    <1%—Special waste, i.e. radioactive, cytotoxic pressurized containers.

11. **When the waste is classified as infectious waste?**

    When the waste contain pathogen of sufficient virulence and quantity as well so that when there is exposure to such waste by a person or animal could eventually result in the infectious disease.

12. **What is the excreted load of enteric disease and infectious agents?**

    As per WHO estimation the excreted load of infectious agents of some of enteric diseases is as under:

Infectious Agent	Average number per gram of feces
Salmonella typhi	10^8
Hepatitis A virus	10^6
Shigella species	10^7
E coli (pathological)	10^8

These organisms in the environment at the temperature of 20–30°C may remain for 2 weeks to 3 months which aggravate the health hazards especially when associated with biomedical waste generated in healthcare facility.

13. **What are the major components of heathcare waste in India?**

Components	Percentage (approx)
Bandages	30–35
Plastic	7–10
Glass	3–5
Disposable syringes	0.3–0.5

14. **What is an average percentage of plastic and paper in hospital waste?**
    Plastic   70%
    Paper   15%

15. **What is hazardous waste?**
    The waste products which by their characteristics poses threat to environment or human life. For example, radioactive waste, pressurized cans, infectious waste, etc.

16. **What is biomedical waste?**
    The waste generated in diagnosis treatment or immunization of human beings or animals, in research or in the production of testing of biological products including all categories of infected and toxic waste that is potential threat to human beings and environment. Biomedical waste can also be termed as regulated waste/medical waste or health care waste.

17. **What is hospital waste?**
    All discarded biological and nonbiological material which is not intended for further use.

18. **How biomedical waste/medical waste is generated?**
    It can be generated during:
    - Diagnosis
    - Treatment
    - Immunization
    - Biomedical research
    - Production and testing of biological products.

19. **What is infectious waste/clinical waste?**
    Waste capable of producing an infectious disease based on four factors namely.
    1. Presence of virulent pathogenic organism
    2. Portal of entry
    3. Sufficient dose of pathogen
    4. Resistance of the host.

20. **What are the characteristics of general waste?**
    It is:
    - Non-hazardous
    - Non-toxic
    - Non-infectious
    - Disposed through local municipal authorities.

21. **Give examples of infectious waste?**
    - Waste from infectious wards
    - Human blood and blood products
    - Cultures and stocks of infectious agents
    - Waste from surgery and autopsy
    - Contaminated sharps
    - Dialysis unit waste
    - Contaminated animal carcasses
    - Contaminated equipments.

22. **What are the hazards of pressurized containers?**
    There may explode if punctured or incinerated and cause damage nearby. They should be returned to manufacturer as far as possible.

23. **What are the indirect risks associated with biomedical waste?**
    The risk associated with biomedical waste per se:
    - Contamination of ground soil and water by dumping untreated waste
    - In case there is insufficient filtering then smoke can pollute the air.

24. **What is net wastivity?**
    It is the net quantity of waste generated in proportion inputs. This excludes the recyclable waste.

25. **How will you calculate the average quantity of waste generated?**
    By using the formula:
    Average quantity of generated per day divided by the bed occupied on that particular day.

26. **How the hospital waste can be classified?**
    It can be classified as follows:
    - As per biomedical waste (management and handling rules 1998), there are 10 categories.
    - As per WHO there are 8 categories.
    - As per environment protection Act of USA there are 7 categories.

27. **Why housekeeping department is "police" of the hospital?**
    P – Planning   O – Organize   L – Liaison
    I – Implementation   C – Control/Monitor   E – Evaluation

28. **What are the categories of waste as per WHO?**
    - General waste
    - Pathological waste
    - Radioactive waste
    - Chemical waste
    - Infectious waste
    - Sharps
    - Pharmaceutical waste
    - Pressurized containers.

29. **What is the quantum of biomedical waste in different countries?**
    The quantum of waste generated per bed per day is:

Country	Quantity (Kg/Bed/Day)
USA	4.5
Spain	3.0
UK	2.5
France	2.5
India	1.5

30. **In India what is the composition of biomedical waste?**
    The composition as per weight is

Waste Type	Percentage (approx.)
Plastic waste	15
Non combustible	22
Wet cellublostic solid *	18
Dry cellublostic solid *	45

    *combustible waste

31. **What is an average quantity of waste per day?**
    It ranges between 1 and 3 kg per day per bed of which 2 kg is incinerable waste.

32. **Name the sources of biomedical waste.**
    - Hospital, nursing homes, clinics, dispensaries
    - Blood banks
    - Industries
    - Household (generates less than .5% of total waste).

33. **What are the waste generated by microbiology laboratory?**
    1. Laboratory cultures
    2. Stocks and/or specimens of microorganisms
    3. Attenuated and/or live vaccines
    4. Human or animal cell cultures which are used in research
    5. Laboratory material which has come into contact with any of the above.

34. **Classify the hospital waste.**

    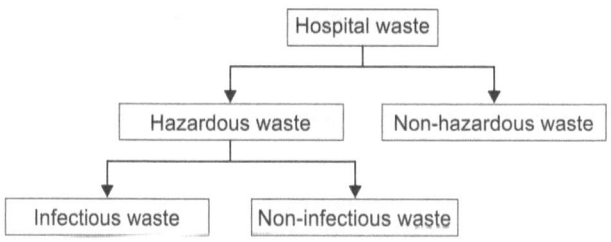

35. **Give examples of biodegradable and non-biodegradable waste.**
    Biodegradable waste: Peel of fruits, paper, vegetable skin, leftover food, etc.
    Non-biodegradable waste: Foils, wrapping plastics, etc.

12 Hospital Waste

36. **Classify the hospital waste in percentage.**
    - Hazardous waste   10–25%
    - Non-hazardous waste   75–90%
    - Infectious waste   15–18%
    - Non-infectious waste   5–7%

37. **What are the types of hazardous waste?**
    a. Injurious
    b. Cytotoxic
    c. Infectious
    d. Chemical.

38. **What are routes through which waste may cause transmission of disease?**
    - Inhalation
    - Absorption
    - Ingestion
    - Injury.

39. **What is the hospital waste which needs special disposal?**
    - Pharmaceuticals waste
    - Radioactive waste (solid, liquid and gaseous)
    - Laboratory waste.

40. **How the radioactive waste is disposed?**
    It is disposed as per the regulations laid down by Atomic Energy Commission (AEC).

41. **How the radiological waste is disposed?**
    - **Solid:** By storage during which its radioactivity is reduced to acceptable level over a period of time or by size reduction in which under controlled condition waste is incinerated and ashes are disposed safely.
    - **Liquid:** By diluting the waste and released into existing sewage system into very small amount over extended period of time.

42. **When the chemical waste is considered hazardous?**
    If the chemical waste is:
    - Corrosive
    - Toxic
    - Genotoxic/cytotoxic
    - Toxic in general
    - Reactive.

43. **Which are the potential toxic waste from hospitals?**
    - Radioactive waste—radiotherapy isotopes
    - Pharmaceutical waste (antibiotics, cytotoxic analgesics, etc.)
    - Chemical waste (disinfectants, reagents, X-ray dark room chemicals).

44. **What effect cytotoxic waste may produce?**
    a. Immune suppression
    b. Cancer
    c. Fetal abnormalities
    d. Pancytopenia
    e. Genetic abnormalities.

45. **What are the diseases biomedical waste can cause?**
    - Tuberculosis
    - Hepatitis B/C
    - HIV/AIDS
    - Gastroenteritis
    - Tetanus
    - Skin injection
    - Typhoid fever (enteric fever)
    - Fetal abnormalities.

46. **Who are the persons at risk of getting infected with biomedical waste (BMW)?**
    - Healthcare workers (doctors, nurses, lab tech, attendants, sweeper, waste handlers, etc.)
    - Patients and their attendants
    - Workers of hospital support services (workers of laundry, waste store room, transportation, etc.)
    - Rag pickers.

47. **What are different steps in health care waste management?**
    These steps can be represented in the form of flowchart (*see on the next page*).

48. **What are the goals of biomedical waste management (BMWM)?**
    - Cost containment by reducing waste
    - Reduction in environmental pollution
    - Protecting community health
    - Reduction in hazards
    - Enhancement of hospital image.

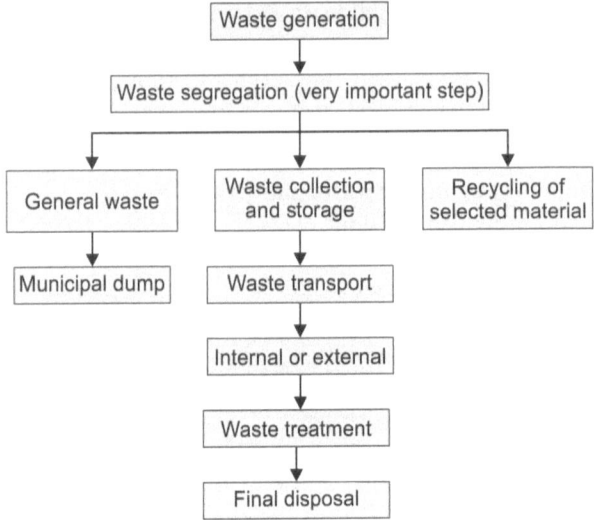

49. **What should be the measures to ensure proper waste management rules?**
    - Regular inspection of the site of BMW generation regarding other steps being followed or not
    - Sufficient supply of the material needed for BMWM
    - Daily record maintenance of incinerator temperature
    - Feedback from staff and people involved in BMWM
    - Periodic communication with central and state pollution control board
    - Training and update to the staff and waste handlers.

50. **Mention the characteristics of the bags used for BMW.**
    - Bags used for incineration should be of non-chlorinated material
    - Bags used for autoclaving should be heat resistant.

51. **What are the main characteristics of the waste?**
    - Compaction characteristics
    - Bulk density
    - Acidity
    - Viscosity
    - Moisture
    - Volatile matter
    - Calorific value

- Ash
- Fixed carbon.

52. **Describe briefly each of characteristic.**
    - *Compaction characteristics:* To what extent the waste can be made compact so as to reduce transport contained dispersal space as volume of waste is reduced considerably. Moisture affects the compaction characteristics adversely.
    - *Bulk density:* It is the weight of a unit volume of a material (gm/cm^3). It is more for all solid waste before treatment and compaction. It is inversely related to the cost of collection and transportation.
    - *Acidity:* pH of waste needs special attention because strong acidic waste are corrosive and reactive and require special treatment to reduce the acidity.
    - *Viscosity:* It is fluidity of the waste and inversely related with temperature, i.e. if temperature increases viscosity decreases this waste become more fluid in nature.
    - *Volatile matter:* The presence of volatile matter in waste which turns into gaseous form on high temperature. This is estimated by heating the waste material in furnace at 200°C for 10 minutes.
    - *Calorific value:* This is the amount of heat released from combustion of unit weight of substance.
    - *Ash contents:* This is amount of ash produced when material is completely burnt. Ash of a material may be toxic or non-toxic and knowledge about composition of ash guides about suitable disposal.
    - *Moisture contents of waste:* This can be estimated by drying the waste at 104–110°C for 24 hours and then weighting and finding the difference in weight before drying and after drying. More moisture content leads to incomplete and low quality boring.
    - *Fixed carbon:* It is the portion of the waste which is left after eliminating moisture and volatile matter excluding ash. It is calculated using the following formula:
    Fixed carbon% = 100 − (Moisture% + Volatile matter%)
    Total carbon = Volatile matter + Fixcd carbon.

53. **What is the linkage between biomedical waste management with municipal waste management?**
    Since health care establishments are located within the municipal area therefore formers waste management has a close linkage

with the municipal system of waste management. Also the civic authority is responsible for public health. For this reason the health care establishments must have a clear and close understanding with the municipality regarding sharing of responsibilities associated with this issue.

Three-fourth of the total hospital waste is not hazardous/infected (provided strict segregation is practised) and can even be taken care of by the municipal waste management system. For example waste generated at the hospital kitchen, garden, office, store, etc.

The practices of strict and careful segregation of waste at the generation site would reduce the load and the cost of management of the actually hazardous and infected biomedical waste at every step of collection, transportation, treatment and final disposal.

For every health care establishment it is not possible to have its own full-fledged waste treatment and disposal system hence the need for common treatment and disposal facilities arises which can be under the ownership/supervision/guidance of the civic authority.

54. **When for the first time the issue of biomedical waste was discussed?**

The issue of biomedical waste was first time discussed in 1983 in Norway at meeting convened by the WHO. The issue was fuelled by the reports of beach washing of medical waste on the coasts of Gulf and Florida state. Another issue was recycling of disposable articles in third world countries because of their sparse resources and weak economy.

55. **What are the role of district level monitoring committee in BMWM rules amendments 2011?**

The district level monitoring committee is established by the government of every state and union territory and will work at district level to monitor compliance by occupier to BMWM rules in healthcare facility as well as in common treatment facility. The chairman of committee is District Medical Officer (DMO).

56. **Why there is need of biomedical waste management in healthcare facility?**

The need of proper management of hospital waste management is felt because of following reasons:

- Injuries from sharps leading to infection to all categories of hospital personnel and waste handler.
- Hospital acquired infections in patients from poor infection control practices among hospital staff and poor waste management by stakeholders.
- Risk of infection outside hospital for waste handlers and scavengers and at time general public living in the vicinity of hospitals.
- Risk associated with hazardous chemicals, drugs to persons handling wastes at all levels.
- "Disposable" discarded in waste without any mutilation being repacked and sold by unscrupulous elements without even being washed.
- Drugs which have been disposed off, being repacked and sold off to unsuspecting buyers.
- Risk of air, water and soil pollution directly due to waste, or due to defective incineration emission and ash.

Chapter 3

Effect of Hospital Waste on Environment and Health

1. **Define macronutrients and micronutrients.**
   Those elements which required in large amount are known as macronutrients while those in very small amount called micronutrients.

2. **What is INSOLATION?**
   It is the combination of words:
   - Incoming
   - Solar
   - Radiation.

3. **How many types of radiation are there from the ground?**
   Terrestrial radiation: These are long waves, low frequency infrared (heat) radiations emitted by earth including its atmosphere. They are the electromagnetic radiations.

   Counter radiation: Redirection of part of the earth's terrestrial radiation back to the surface due to green house effect.

4. **What is green house effect?**
   This is the natural phenomena to keep the earth temperature balanced by virtue of trapping heat energy.
   This can be produced artificially in house by using glass, which acts as a barrier.

5. **How hospital wastes contribute to green house effect?**
   Due to emission of methane gas, which is a natural byproduct of decomposition of solid waste, from landfills. By reducing the amount of landfill solids the emission can be reduced and in turn the green house effects.

6. **What is the advantage of green house effect?**
   Because of trapping of heat energy by green house gases (water vapor, carbon dioxide, methane, nitrous oxide, chlorofluorocarbon, ozone, etc.) the earth surface is warmer, (mean temperature 15°C) and comfortable. Had this effect not been there the average temperature could have gone below zero degree (mean temperature –19°C). Due to increase in green house gas there is already increase in global temperature.

7. **Why health care waste became hazardous?**
   Because of following reasons:
   - It may contain infectious or radioactive agent
   - It may contain sharp
   - It may be genotoxic
   - It may contain hazardous chemicals.

8. **How the risk from unmanaged biomedical waste can pose to general population?**
   The general population can be affected in three ways:
   1. Exposure to chemical pollutants like dioxin and mercury from incineration of the waste
   2. Accidental exposure from contact with waste at municipal waste disposal bins
   3. Exposure to biological or chemical contaminants in water.

9. **What is the approximate time to degenerate various types of waste generated by human activity?**
   The type of litter genterated by human activities and approximate time taken in ascending order for degeneration is as follows:

Waste product	Approximate time for degeneration
Organic waste (fruits and vegetable peels, leftover food stuff)	1–2 weeks
Paper	10–30 days
Cotton cloth	2–5 months
Woolen items	One year
Wood	10–15 years
Tin, aluminum and cans made of metals	100–500 years
Plastics bags	One million years
Glass products	Undetermined

10. **What is the source of green house gases?**
 These gases comes out from natural sources and human activity like, fuel use, industrial growth incinaration of waste. The carbon dioxide is the main green house gas and its residence time is about 230 years and it has been noted that its concentration on 280 ppm of preindustrial era has been increased to 360 ppm.

11. **Which causes the green house effect?**
 The infrared radiations (heat) which when reflected back towards space from earth surface. This heat is absorbed by green house gases (Fig. 3.1).

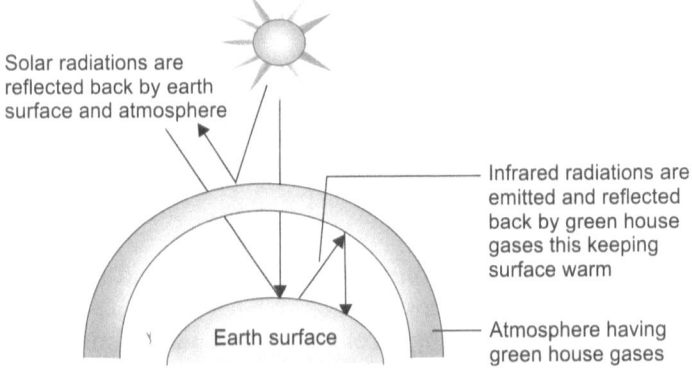

Fig. 3.1: Green house effect.

12. **Why the level of green house gases is increasing?**
 Due to imbalance between emission and absorption of these gases in the atmosphere.

13. **What is environmental pollution?**
 This is an undesirable and excessive addition of the substances to water, land and air thus adversely altering natural quality of the environment. This can be defined as alterations of the natural environment that are harmful to life.
 According to Katyal and Satake, it is the unfavorable alteration of our surroundings wholly or largely as a byproduct of man's action, through direct or indirect effects of changes in energy patterns, radiation levels, chemical and physical constitution and abundance of organisms.

14. **What is pollutant?**
    It is the wrong constituent; in wrong amount at wrong time or wrong place.

15. **What do you understand by primary pollutants and secondary pollutants?**
    Primary pollutants: These are the pollutants which are produced due to direct natural or atmospheric activity. These pollutants do not undergo any chemical change.
    Secondary pollutants: These are the pollutants which are formed due to chemical reactions of primary pollutants and other chemical or physical constituents present in the atmosphere.

16. **How the pollutants are categorized broadly?**
    - Chemical
    - Biological
    - Physical (energy)
    - Radiological.

17. **Describe local and global pollutants.**
    Local pollutants: These are the substances whose concentration cross the threshold concentration within small area or volume of water, land (soil) or air, e.g. house, place of work, etc.
    Global pollutants: Global pollutants are those substances whose concentration level over years have cumulative built up in water, soil, or air, e.g. global warming, ozone depletion (ozone hole).

18. **Can pollution be eliminated?**
    No, it cannot be eliminated completely however, can be reduced to great extent because pollution of any kind is the result of human activity and this cannot be eliminated so the pollution.

19. **How will you describe point source and non-point source pollution?**
    - Point source pollution is a single, identifiable localized source of pollution.
    - Non-point source pollution is different non-identifiable, diffuse source of pollution both the type effect the water, soil, and air (Fig. 3.2).

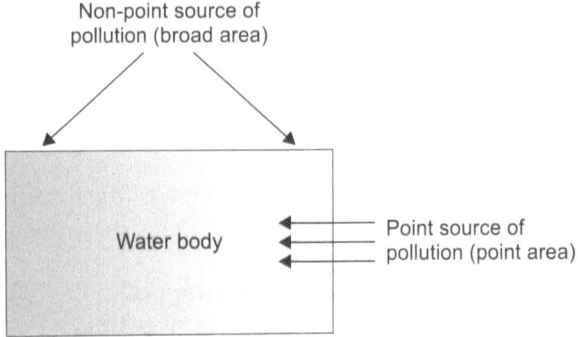

Fig. 3.2: Point and non-point source of pollution.

20. **Give examples of point and non-point source pollution.**
    Point source pollution:
    - Industry/hospital waste water discharge outlet
    - Noise of jet engine
    - Smoke from incinerator

    Non-point source pollution:
    - Sediments
    - Bacteria
    - Nitrogen.

21. **What is water pollution?**
    It is any chemical or physical change in water mainly due to human activities that restricts its use by human being and other live forms.

22. **What is leaching and leachate?**
    Leaching: It is the process in which chemicals from the material dissolves into water while it is being filtered through that material. The resulting mixture is called **leachate** which is consisting of residues from decomposed organic matter and material (Fig. 3.3).

23. **What are the sources of water pollution?**
    - Sewage
    - Industrial waste
    - Biomedical waste
    - Physical pollutants

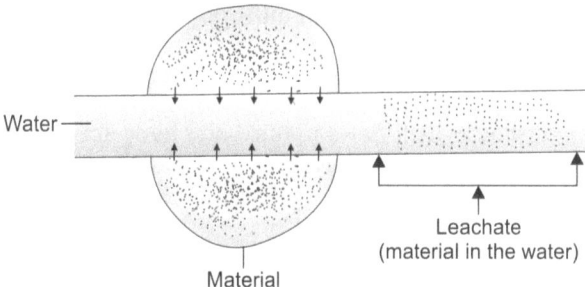

Fig. 3.3: Process of leaching.

- Agricultural pollutants
- Poor land filling leading to leachate.

24. **What are the agents causing water pollution?**
    - **Physical agents:** Insoluble particles of silt and soil.
    - **Chemical agents:**
        - **Organic:** Oil, animal and human manure
        - **Inorganic:** Heavy metals, nitrates, phosphates, acid, etc.
        - **Radioactive substances.**
        - **Biological agents:** Bacteria, virus, protozoa and worm.

25. **Describe eutrophication.**
    It is the process of increase in chemical nutrients (phosphate, nitrate) in water body's ecosystem and results in increasing it's productivity.

    By this process there would be growth of plankton which will consume all dissolved oxygen of that water body thus making water unsuitable for life of fishes and other aquatic animals as water because hypoxic and stagnation of lack.

26. **What are the effects of eutrophication?**
    - Reduction in resource value of water
    - Economic loss
    - Health problem if such water is consumed.

27. **Eutrophication results from:**
    - Nutrient pollution like sewage effluent, runoff lawn fertilizers
    - Natural accumulation
    - Human activities.

28. **Which is the main culprit for eutrophication?**
    Phosphorous is often regarded as the main culprit.

29. **What do mean by algae boom?**
    The nutrients which flows to the water body acts as fertilizers leading to population explosion of algae and this process is called algae boom and this results in green colors of the water body.

30. **How the foaming is caused in water supplies?**
    Due to presence of oil, greasy material and other organic material in the water flow where, it is disturbed or agitated the bubbles form and remain for sometime then eventually burst. These bubbles are formed because of dissolved organic compounds which in turn formed due to metabolism of aquatic organisms.

31. **Write the effects of plant nutrients (phosphates and nitrates).**
    - Algae boom
    - Fish death
    - Upsetting of aquatic ecosystem
    - Eutrophication
    - Toxic for live stock
    - Foul odor.

32. **How thermal pollution of water is caused?**
    This is caused by re-entry of the heat laden water into water body.

33. **What do you understand by thermal pollution of water?**
    When the water which is used from the water body is used by industries for cooling purpose and when this heat laden water goes back to the water body results in the increase in temperature of the water.

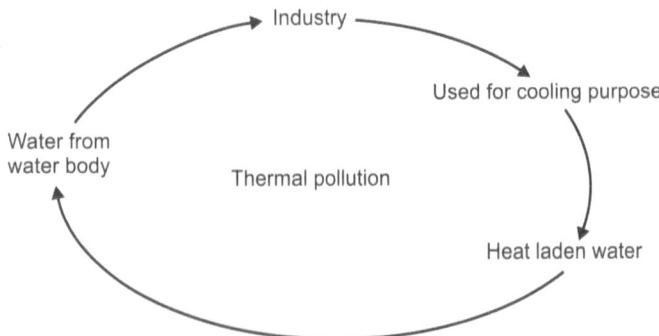

34. What are the sources of land pollution by biomedical waste?
- Infectious waste
- Discarded chemicals and medicines
- Incinerator waste
- Heavy metals (Cd, Pb, Hg) present in waste
- Leachate from landfills.

35. What is land pollution?
It is the addition of undesirable matter to the land that damages the terrestrial organisms, reduces the uses of the land by man for agricultural, recreational, residential purposes and increases the risk of health hazard.

36. What are the international recommendations for waste management?
- Minimization of waste production
- Recycle and reuse the waste to the maximum possible limit
- Choose safe and environment friendly options for waste treatment.
- Careful final disposal of waste in confined and designated land fill area.

37. What are the general principles of BMW management?
These principles are followed by all stakeholders who are involved in BMW management.
- Do no harm to anyone who comes in contact with such waste this is achieved by safe collection, segregation, treatment and disposal of the waste.
- Encouraging use of nondisposable items instead of disposable items because they are environment friendly and their safety are used if they are properly sterilized.
- Following 3 'R' Principle (Reduce, Recycle, Reuse) so as to minimize the waste
- Well monitored and supervised flow of biomedical waste (life cycle approach).

38. What are the benefits of waste minimization?
- Occupational safety
- Financial profit to hospital
- Environmental protection.

39. Mention the various steps which are involved in waste minimization.
- Good purchase procedure to reduce waste
- Composting of organic waste
- Use of recyclable sharp
- More use of biodegradable products
- Follow FIFO principle (First in First out) that means consume the oldest items first
- Strict check on inventory to maintain it optimum
- Adopting procedures for recovery for mercury, lead, silver, etc.
- Recycling of the hospital waste papers
- Purchase of multiple use product and in bulk
- Use item before its expiry.

40. Draw waste cycle diagram.

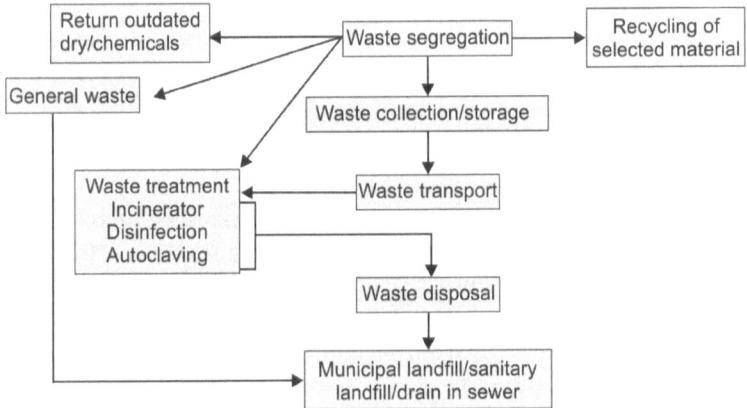

41. What are persistent organic pollutants (POPs)?
The POPs are global treat to environment and because of their chemical stability they stay and accumulate in environment and living organisms for an extended period of time (years or decades). In initial list of 12 POPs were more commonly referred as dirty dozen divided into 3 categories:
1. Pesticides
2. Industrial chemicals
3. Unintended byproducts.

42. What are the characteristics of dioxins?
- They are unintended byproduct of human activities.
- These are also known as repeat offenders

- Fat soluble
- Persistent organic pollutants
- Very stable chemical structure
- Half life is about seven years and tend to bioaccumulate in food chain so high in food chain more concentration of dioxin
- Dioxins are strong adsorbent to soil and degrade by photo-degradation.
- In soil dioxins tend to remain near surface and move towards water bodies through soil erosion and get bioaccumulated in aquatic life.

43. **What are the sources of dioxins?**
    - Industrial processes
    - Forest fire
    - Volcanic eruptions
    - Thermal processing of product like smelting
    - Incinerators giving incomplete combustion
    - Effluent discharge from paper mills that use chlorine bleaching.

44. **What are the effects of short-term and long-term exposure to dioxin effects of short-term exposure?**
    - Skin lesions
    - Attend liver functions
    - Long-term exposure impaired immune, endocrine and reproductive system or

    What is the chemical structure of dioxin and furan (Fig. 3.4)?

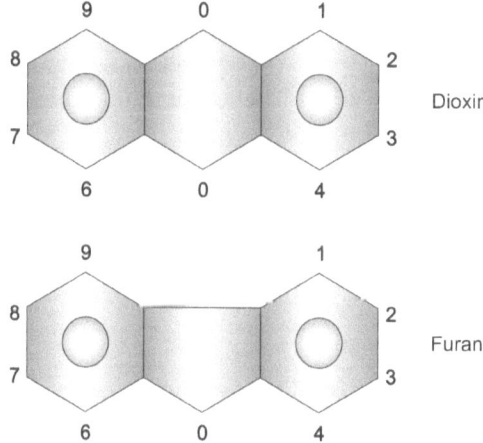

Fig. 3.4: Chemical structure.

Dioxins and furan contain chlorine atoms located at position 1-4 and 6-9. There are 75 different dioxin congeners and 135 different furan congeners.

45. What is the major toxicity of dioxin and furan?

They have been implicated as potential endocrine disrupters as they can interfere with normal functions of hormones and thus affect reproductive success.

46. What are the qualities of environment friendly product?

These products are:
- Creating minimum pollution
- With high recyclable contents
- Less toxic
- With less packing materials
- More energy efficient
- Safer for patients, stuff and environment.

47. How dioxin and furan are formed?

Dioxins and furans are family of polycyclic aromatic hydrocarbons and formed when chlorinated plastic or any chlorine containing material is burnet in presence of organic material. Chlorine molecules get combined with organic matter to form dioxin and furan and the presence of heavy metal acts as catalyst for this chemical process.

48. What is DEHP?

Diethylhexyl phthalate (DEHP): It is a chemical compound which is added to PVC to make the item flexible, moldable and strong. The ratio of PVC with DEHP is 80-60 : 20-40.

It does not bind with PVC hence leach out from PVC products during medical interventions.

49. What are the adverse effects of DEHP?

- Suppressed ovulation
- Reduced liver and kidney functions
- Bradycardia
- Respiratory distress
- Testicular damage.

50. How adverse effect of DEPH be eliminated?

Use nonDEPH products.

51. **How waste causes indirect risk to environment and public health?**

    By:
    - Contamination of water and air due to indiscriminate disposal and burning of waste in open.
    - If waste is disposed in pit which is near water then leachate and contaminate the water thus causing public health problem.

52. **How improper BMW spread the infection?**
    - Through vectors (housefly, mosquito, insects)
    - Through injury or contact with infectious material
    - Through unauthorized recycling of infectious material
    - Through improper use of discarded medicines
    - Through sharp injuries
    - Through indiscriminate disposal of incinerator ash/residue
    - Toxic emersion from improper burning of waste.

53. **What is the impact of biomedical waste on human and environmental health?**

Type of waste	Impact
Anatomical waste	Infections get transmitted through either direct contact or vectors
Laboratory cultures, specimen, vaccines and live microorganisms	Various health disorders like cough, eye redness and burning, skin burn, skin itching, dermatitis are caused when non-treated waste comes in contact
Blood, body fluids, cotton swabs, bandages	Transmission of infections like hepatitis, tuberculosis, enteric fever, and AIDS, etc. either through vectors or by direct contacts
Waste sharps (scalpel, needles, broken glasses, blades)	Transmission of infections like tetanus, hepatitis, septicemia, AIDS, etc. by direct innoculations
Catheters and plastic tubing, PVC surgical gloves	Dissolution of DHEP chemical from PVC material may serve as human carcinogens and may disturb hormonal function in person in close contact

Contd...

Contd...

Type of waste	Impact
IV fluid bottles, blood collection bags & urine-bags	On incineration these products release dioxin and furan, suspended particulate matter, and gases. These articles may get illegally recycled and further aid to spread of infection
Chemical waste (used in disinfections process)	Causes cough, and headache on exposure, on prolong reaction in human body affects normal function of hormones and acts as carcinogens
Cytotoxic chemical waste like anticancer drugs, phenyl, strong alkalis and acids, radioactive materials	Cytotoxic effect can be manifested in the form of fetal abnormalities, skin diseases, ulcers, cancer and anemia
Incineration ash	Partially incinerated ash may be source of various infections

54. **What are the environmental problems arised from disposal of untreated biomedical waste?**

    Following are environmental problems which arise from disposal of untreated biomedical waste:
    - Decomposing of waste may generate foul and obnoxious odor in the healthcare facility premises or surrounding area.
    - Waste dumps may attract stray animals and birds that will spread the untreated waste material leading to unhygienic and unaesthetic environment.
    - Waste may clog the drainage system leading to unhygienic surrounding environment and may act as breading grounds from flies and mosquitoes which further spread the disease.
    - The ground water may get contaminated by formation of leachate from untreated decomposing waste.
    - Disastrous ecological effects may be produced by contamination of ground water and land by indiscriminate disposal of pharmaceutical waste.
    - Open burning or uncontrolled incineration of waste can generate dioxin and furan gases which causes air pollution.

55. **What is the advantages of having air pollution control unit along with incinerator?**

    Because the biomedical waste contains high percentage of chlorine in the form of disinfectants or plastics (PVC) and incineration of these material produces dioxin which enters environment as fumes. Installation of air pollution control units help in concentrating dioxin in the form of fly ash which is fine solid and removed from the flue stack.

56. **Why the problem of environmental pollution is more in third world countries?**

    The problem of environmental pollution which started with the advent of the human being on Earth has now reached to extremely dangerous level both in developed and developing places. As the fact of loss of self-cleaning capacity of the air, developed countries already woken up and laid down stringent safety standards and measures to maintain the power of the balance of nature in the area of waste management, particularly in the area of biomedical waste management. However the developing (third world) countries were lagging behind in laying down stringent norms for waste management resulting in pollution problems, which is very harmful, detrimental or injurious to public health.

57. **What is the reason for environmental disruption in developing countries.**

    Because of growth is industrial production there is adverse effects on natural environment which disturbed balance of nature. The capability of self-maintenance and self-regulation of system has been disrupted by the continuous uncontrolled discharge of variety of industrial pollutants. Moreover, improper treatment and discharge of waste and its unhygienic disposal in natural resources has created a serious problem for biotic and abiotic components of the environment.

Chapter 4

Generation and Segregation

1. **What is the average quantity of waste per day?**
   In India an average quantity of waste generated in between 0.5 and 2 kg whereas in developed countries this quantity may range from 3 to 10 kg because of excessive use of disposable items. India has around 6,88,160 beds this producing 876.72 tones of waste per day.

2. **How the biomedical waste is quantified on per patient bed per day basis?**
   The biomedical waste is quantified by using formula
   Total quantum of waste generated per day (w) divided by total number of patient beds occupied at a time (B)
   $$Q = W/B$$

3. **Mention the items contained in solid waste generated in hospital.**
   Various items are contained the solid waste in hospital and segregation is important as by this procedure infectious waste content is reduced to considerable limit.
   Contents of solid waste are:
   - Bandages, linen, etc.
   - Disposable plastic syringes
   - Plastic and papers
   - General waste including food, fruit and vegetable peels
   - Other waste.

4. What are the major components of healthcare waste in Indian?

Components	Percentage (approx)
Bandages	30–35
Plastic	7–10
Glass	3–5
Disposable syringes	0.3–0.5

5. What type of waste is generated in operation theater?
   - Anatomical waste
   - Cotton, bandages
   - Liquid waste
   - Sharps

6. Mention the waste types generated in laboratory.
   - Microbiology waste
   - Liquid waste
   - Sharps

7. What are the sources of liquid waste generation in hospital?
   The sources for liquid waste in hospital:
   - Laboratory
   - Laundry
   - Housekeeping activities
   - Disinfecting activities
   - Cleaning
   - Washing

8. Can chemical liquid waste be mixed with other waste?
   No, in no circumstance chemical liquid waste be mixed with other hospital waste but there should be separate collection system which is leading to effluent treatment system.

9. How many types of X-ray waste is generated?
   There are four types of wastes generated during X-ray procedure:
   1. X-ray fixer
   2. X-ray developer
   3. X-ray cleaner
   4. X-ray lead shields/foils

10. **What is the percentage of plastic in hospital solid waste?**
    It is around 8-12% and if use of plastic is not restricted then it may increase further.

11. **Why so much plastic items used in hospital?**
    This is because of qualities of plastic which are:
    - Transparency
    - High resale value in market
    - Single use (disposable)
    - Low cost
    - Low infection rate because of single use.

12. **Name the plastics which are in common use in hospital item.**
    - PVC – poly vinyl chloride
    - PET – Polyethylene terephthalate
    - Polyamide
    - Polyethylene
    - Polycarbonate
    - Polyeruptylene
    - Polyurethrane.

13. **Why plastic (PVC) containers should not be used for solution?**
    As PVC contains lead cadmium and phthalate which may slowly leach into the contained solution and cause toxicity on prolonged use.

14. **What happens when PVC item is burned?**
    It produces furans and dioxins which are known for causing various health problems like:
    - Cancer
    - Allergies
    - Disturbances in liver enzymes
    - Depression in body immune system
    - Teratogenecity.

15. **What is the best solution for plastic nuisance?**
    Minimize plastic use which can be achieved through following practices:
    - Use material when absolute necessary
    - Replace disposable item with more conventional and reusable item
    - Purchase ecofriendly material/items
    - Buy in bulk so as to reduce the making materials which sometimes contain plastics.

16. **How effectively waste can be collected in bags for segregation?**
    - Specified color bag should be fixed in containers
    - Waste should not spill out of bag
    - There should be no mixing of infectious and non-infectious waste
    - Bag should be removed from container when it is ¾ filled and tied so that waste does not spill out
    - Needle should be destroyed first by needle destroyer and head of syringe be mutilated
    - Plastic items should be disinfected with 1% hypochlorite solution for 30 min contact period
    - Containers and bags should bear biohazard symbol.

17. **Define segregation.**
    It is the process of segregation of different types of waste as per their treatment and disposal option.

18. **What is the minimum thickness of plastic bag used to collect the waste?**
    55 micron thickness (high density polythene).

19. **On what factors does effective segregation depends?**
    - Type of hospital/institution
    - Motivation of the hospital staff
    - Training of the staff
    - Health care waste management of the hospital.

20. **What is the main purpose of segregation?**
    To separate different categories of hospital waste [as per biomedical waste management (BMWM) and handling rule 1998] and place it in different containers/bags. It is the key to effective BMWM.

21. **What should be the characteristics of the containers?**
    They should be of:
    - Appropriate size
    - Smooth inside lining
    - Well rounded
    - Well labeled
    - Not too heavy
    - Easily handled by one person
    - Can be cleaned and disinfected easily
    - Foot operated lid.

22. **On what factor does choice of size of container depend?**
    a. Frequency of collection
    b. Expected amount of waste.

23. **Write basic principles of segregation.**
    a. Elimination of segregation at waste disposal site
    b. Reduction in volume of waste to be treated
    c. Maintain safety standards for workers
    d. Facilitation of recycling process.

24. **Which is the best place of waste segregation?**
    At the sites of waste generation, i.e. ward, OT, lab, clinic, etc. because here it becomes simple and cost effective, less harming and responsibility lies with the generator like doctor, nurse, technician, etc.

25. **Mention the principles through which effective segregation can be achieved.**
    - By education and training of the staff (generator and waste handlers)
    - Placement of proper color coded bins at place of generation
    - Regular identification of waste composition
    - Developing simple and realistic goals and targets
    - Effective regular communication between generator, handler and contractors
    - Proper coding and labeling of waste bins
    - Making effective work environment and making suitable changes in work practices
    - Make the segregation single stage, i.e. the segregated material remains in the same beg during collection, storage, transport and disposal.

26. **What are the benefits of effective segregation?**
    - Improved infection control
    - Protection of staff from infectious diseases
    - Proper disposal of waste and reduce hazards
    - Establish uniform waste management practices among staff
    - Cost reduction
    - Training of the staff
    - Enhanced image of hospital
    - Effective plan should be simple and time efficient.

27. **Why generator of the waste is responsible for the segregation?**
    This is because the generator (doctor, nurse and technician) are aware of that:
    - Material is infectious
    - Material is hazardous
    - Used material is sharp and can cause injury
    - They are wearing proper protective equipment
    - They have already handled the waste.

28. **Why the responsibility of segregation lies with waste generator?**
    This is because of the following reasons:
    1. Waste generator know exactly what material has been used.
    2. S/he has already used the material before and knows its importance.
    3. Waste generator is equipped with personal protective equipment (PPE) at the time of waste generation.
    4. S/he know the type of item that was used on whether on infectious patient or laboratory experiments.
    5. Patient caregiver knows exactly which cytotoxic, pharmaceutical or chemical was used.
    6. S/he know what material was used during patient care or diagnostic procedures.
    7. Waste generator is well trained person in biomedical waste handling.

29. **Make flowchart of segregation and recycling of nonhazardous health care waste.**

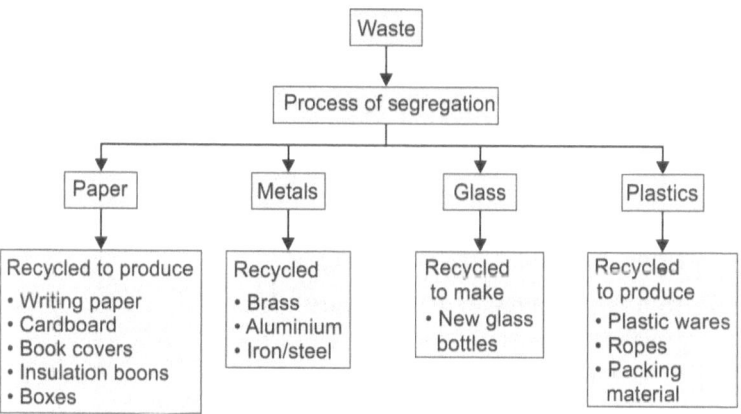

Generation and Segregation

30. **What are the advantages of segregation?**
    a. General waste does not become infectious
    b. Total cost of waste treatment is lowered
    c. Reduction in chances of infecting health care workers.

31. **What percentage of hospital waste is nonhazardous?**
    50-80% waste is nonhazardous and can be disposed off easily.

32. **Where is the pretreatment of segregated waste done?**
    At the site of generation of waste.

33. **What are the advantages of pretreatment of the waste?**
    a. To make recyclable items unusable
    b. To meet obligation of BMW rules
    c. To disinfect the waste so it is no longer infectious.

34. **How the general waste is segregated?**
    - Waste which will go for composting
    - Waste that will go to landfill
    - Waste which can be recycled like paper
    - Cardboard, glass, aluminum cans, etc.

35. **Write about color coding of containers for waste segregation.**
    Yellow   -   Waste category 1, 2, 3, 6
    Red   -   Category 3, 6, 7
    Blue/transparent white -   Category 4, 7
    Black   -   Waste category 5, 9, 10.
    - Category 8 and 10 do not require any container
    - Category 3 is disinfected locally and need not be put in container.

36. **What are the benefits of color coding?**
    - Assistance in proper segregation of waste
    - Identification of hazardous and infectious waste so that staff is aware.
    - Marking segregated waste for prescribed treatment and disposal required.
    - Identification of the waste in bags.

37. **Mention advantages of using plastic bags.**
    - Easy transportation of waste
    - Spillage preventions
    - Waste is out of site of view of patients and visitors
    - Original container remains always clean.

38. **What precautions should be used while using plastic bags?**
    - Plastic bags should not be reused
    - Bag should not be over filled
    - Sharp should not be collected in ordinary plastic bags
    - Red colored bag should not be sent for incineration
    - Bags should be stored secured and inaccessible to animals.

39. **What are the characteristics of waste containers?**
    Container should be:
    - Leak proof
    - Rigid
    - Puncture resistant
    - Foot operated lids
    - Non-reactive to any of the biomedical waste substance which are put in these containers.

40. **What should be main characteristics of reusable waste containers?**
    These are as below:
    - Reusable waste containers must be made of metal or rigid plastic.
    - These containers would be able to withstand exposure to common cleaning materials.
    - Containers must be color codes accordingly so there is no mixing of waste at the site of generation.
    - The containers must be labeled with the biohazard symbol.
    - There should be no leak or holes in containers and label should be clear and updated.

41. **When the container should be cleaned?**
    As soon as possible the leak or spill is observed within the container. This is done for two reasons one is to prevent odors and second exposure of the staff to any infectious material.

42. **What care should be taken in case of sharp containers.**
    The main points for care are:
    - The container should be located near the point of use so as to avoid carrying exposed sharp to significant distance.
    - The container should never be filled more than ¾ of its capacity in order to prevent sharp injuries due to overfilling.
    - The containers should be preferably foot operated.

- Sharp container should never have flap lid
- The sharp waste should never be forcibly be pushed in to the containers.

43. **What problems may arise with the disinfectant material placed in sharp containers?**
    Following may arise from the liquid in sharp containers:
    - The disinfectant solution may not be in contact with all the sharp waste place in container resulting in deficient degree of decontamination.
    - It may pose hazard for contact for staff with aerosols and sharp objects.
    - The liquid may get spilled if the container is toppled for any reason.

44. **Can a second hand or used container be used as sharp containers?**
    Yes, the used container can be used as sharp container if the container is approved by concerned official authorized to certify for such use.

45. **What type of container will be for blue category waste?**
    The container will be cardboard box with blue colored marking.

46. **What type of waste will be collected in blue container?**
    (1) Glassware: Broken or discarded and contaminated glass including medicine vials and ampoules except those contaminated with cytotoxic wastes.
    (2) Metallic body implants

47. **What type of container will be for white category waste?**
    The container should be translucent, puncture proof, leak proof and temper proof.

48. **What type of waste will be collected in white container?**
    The waste which is collected in white container are needles, syringes with fixed needles, needle tip collected from needle cutter or burner, scalpels, blades or other discarded and contaminated metallic sharp which may accidently cause puncture.

49. **What categories of biomedical waste is collected in yellow bin.**
    - **Human anatomical waste:** Human tissues, organs, body parts and fetus, below the viability period.

- **Animal anatomical waste:** Experimental animal carcasses, body parts, organs, tissues, including the waste generated from animals used in experiments or testing in veterinary hospitals or colleges or animal houses.
- **Soiled waste:** Items contaminated with blood, body fluids like dressings, plaster casts, cotton swabs and bags containing residual or discarded blood and blood components.
- **Expired or discarded medicines:** Pharmaceutical waste like antibiotics, cytotoxic drugs including all items contaminated with cytotoxic drugs along with glass or plastic ampoules, vials, etc.
- **Chemical waste:** Chemicals used in production of biological and used or discarded disinfectants.
- **Chemical liquid waste:** Liquid waste generated due to use of chemicals in production of biological and used or discarded disinfectants, silver X-ray film developing liquid, discarded formalin, infected secretions, aspirated body fluids, liquid from laboratories and floor washings, cleaning, house-keeping and disinfecting activities, etc.
- **Discarded linen, mattresses, beddings** contaminated with blood or body fluid.
- **Microbiology, biotechnology and other clinical laboratory waste:** Blood bags, laboratory cultures, stocks or specimens of microorganisms, live or attenuated vaccines, human and animal cell cultures used in research, industrial laboratories, production of biological, residual toxins, dishes and devices used for cultures.

50. **What categories of biomedical waste is collected in red bin?**

    This class of waste is also known as recyclable waste. The waste which come under this category are wastes generated from disposable items such as tubing, bottles, intravenous tubes and sets, catheters, urine bags, syringes (without needles and fixed needle syringes and vacutainers with their needles cut) and gloves.

51. **How the requirement of bags calculated for 200 bedded hospital?**

Waste generated per bed	- 1 kg
Total waste generated	- 200 kg
If one bag can accommodate waste	- 10 kg

Generation and Segregation

Total no. of bags needed	-	(20) bags
If there is improper segregation of infected waste then % of infected waste	-	50-60%
Then no. of yellow bags needed	-	(10-12) bags
If there is proper segregation of waste then	-	10-15%
% of infected waste	-	1-2 bags
% of plastic waste with strict segregation	-	5%
	-	1-2 bags
For general waste no. of bags needed	-	(6-8)

52. **Which is the ideal bin for collecting the biomedical waste?**
    Characteristics of an ideal bin for waste collection are:
    - It should be foot operated so there no hand touch to the waste
    - It should have proper color as prescribed in rules
    - Its rim should be such that the liner can be placed snuggly fitted
    - The size of the bin should corroborate with the quantum of waste generated in the area/unit.
    - It should be nonperforated.

53. **Does the responsibility of healthcare facility occupier ends once the waste is handed over to the common waste treatment facility provider?**
    No, the healthcare facility provider is responsible for any negligence eased by common waste facility provider in waste collection, transportation, treatment or final disposal of the waste belonging to that particular occupier.

54. **Can waste be minimized?**
    Yes, biomedical waste can be minimized to considerable extent by:
    - By avoiding source reduction, i.e. avoiding wastage.
    - Whenever and wherever possible use sterilizable reusable items
    - Segregation of biomedical waste at point of generation of waste
    - Strict control over inventory so that there is wastage due to spoilage of items like drugs, blood, IV fluids, etc.
    - Making appropriate changes in the purchase policy so more non PVC items are purchased.

55. **Is labeling of containers/bags essential?**
    Yes

56. **Why?**
    Labeling of containers of bags in transport vehicle ensures safe and efficient transfer of waste from point of generation to treatment area thus reducing the risk of injuring.

57. **What are the specifications of labeling?**
    - Biohazard to be placed on containers having infectious/pathological waste.
    - Cytotoxic hazard to be placed on cytotoxic waste.
    - Recommended size of symbol and wards to be 80 mm.
    - Labels should be made of permanent marker, so that does not get washed off on cleaning of container.

Chapter 5

Transport and Storage

1. **Define waste transportation.**
   It is the process of carrying away the segregated waste from point of generation to the site of its treatment and disposal.
   Waste can be transported to on-site or off-site storage and treatment area.

2. **What are the components of transport chain?**
   - Point of generation
   - Nursing station
   - Kerb collection point
   - Waste storage area
   - Treatment area

3. **Give the types of the waste transport.**
   There are two types of waste transport:
   1. Within the health care facility known as internal or intramural transport
   2. Outside the health care facility known as external or extramural transport.

4. **Give brief account of intramural and extramural transport.**

   Intramural transport: If the transport of waste from the point of generation to the place where it is temporarily stored before taking for final treatment and disposal.

   Extramural transport: This is the transport of the waste from temporary storage area to the final treatment and disposal.

5. **Name the vehicles for transport of waste.**
   Vehicles for internal transport:
   - **Waste trolley:** It has inbuilt component in which segregated bags of waste are kept.
   - **Push cart:** This is four wheeled cart having side railings and in the middle of cart space is available to keep big containers. Cart may accommodate 2–3 bins.

   Vehicles for external transport:
   - **Cycle rickshaw:** It is used by the institutions where disposal site is nearby. It should be covered from all sides and secured on top.
   - **Van or waste lorry:** It is the collection vehicle—generally used for off site (TWF) transportation of waste. It has biohazard symbol and biomedical waste labeling along with telephone number of the treatment facility owner.

6. **What care should be taken while transporting the waste?**
   - Waste bag should be properly tied and labeled (Fig. 5.1)
   - Bag should be picked up by the neck and placed straight vertical so that it is again picked up by neck only

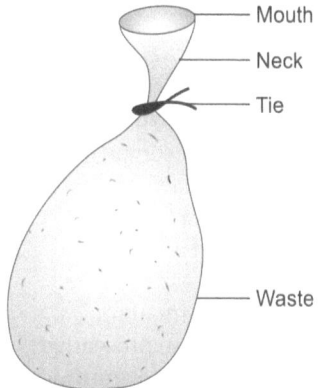

Fig. 5.1: Waste bag.

   - Waste bag/container should not be thrown or dropped
   - Pick up one bag at a time
   - Handling of the bag should be minimal to avoid needle prick injury

- During transportation segregated bags should be kept in designated compartment or area or container
- Waste should be routed through predestinated and shortest route and this route should not be changed
- Vehicle being used for waste transportation should not be used for any other purpose
- Bags should not be handled till securely tied
- After removing the bag container should be properly cleaned and disinfected
- If lift is being used for waste transportation then it should be reserved for this purpose only
- Waste should not spill during transportation
- For internal transport the route should be such that it is not being used by public and should be transported when there is minimum movement in the health care facility
- The waste handler transporting the waste should use the protective gear while transporting
- Waste should not be mixed while transporting
- Hand should not be put into the bags.

7. **What is on-site transportation?**

   It is the transportation of waste from the point of generation to final waste storage area in the hospital itself.

8. **Mention the qualities of the trolley used for waste transport.**
   - Trolley or cart should be reserved for waste transportation only
   - It should not have any sharp projection or corners
   - It should be easy to clean
   - It should be easy to load and unload
   - Trolley/cart should be easy to move
   - It should be maintained regularly
   - Vehicle handler should use protective gear
   - Trolley should be able to accommodate 3 big containers—yellow, red and black.

9. **What are the protective gears?**
   - Cap
   - Mask
   - Heavy duty rubber gloves
   - Plastic apron
   - Gum boots.

10. **What are the best practices for personal protection and rationale behind them?**

Best practices are professional procedures that are accepted or prescribed as being the most effective. In case of BMWM following are the best practices for waste management.

Best Practice 1—wear sterile gloves, masks, apron, shoes and eye protectors while working in laboratory, operation theater and labor room.

Rationale: These protective equipment will protect during procedure and/or patient care, from the exposure to blood, body fluids and other aerosols which may contain infectious pathogens like HBV, HIV, HCV, etc. The protective equipments will act as barrier and prevent cross infections.

Use gloves while touching blood, body fluids, secretions, excretions, also while touching non intact skin (ulcers) and mucous membrane.

Best Practice 2—manage sharp waste carefully with use of needle destroyer and sharp containers.

Rationale: It has been studied and noted that 5% of needlestick injuries occur while recapping, 15% during disposal and 40% after use or before disposal. The effects of needlestick varies depending on whether needle was solid or hollow body in which latter is more dangerous because of amount of blood present in it. It is to note that needlestick injuries are responsible for 40-60% of HBV and HCV infection in hospital workers. The advantage of needle destroyer is that it mitigates the chances of needle reuse and recapping. Another advantage is that it reduces the quantum of sharp waste.

Best Practice 3—do not mix the biomedical waste.

Rationale: Mixing of biomedical waste with general waste leads to potential health hazards to waste handler who may not take enough precautions while dealing with general waste. The mixing of general and potentially infectious waste may also lead to environmental pollution and community health problem at large.

Best Practices 4—Immunization of healthcare workers against HBV.

Rationale: Healthcare workers are vulnerable to get infected to mild to serious infections while giving care to patients or from work place environment. Immunization ensures safety from these occupational hazards. The prevention is always easy, faster, cheaper than cure. Infection prevention to the staff reduces the extra financial burden on organization for treatment of infection contracted.

Best Practices 5— do not store biomedical waste for long periods in the hospital premises.

Rationale: Due to long storage time (beyond 48 hours) there are chances that noninfected waste may become infected waste. During prolonged storage waste many attract rodents and other animals and other nonauthorized people who may incidentally get infected.

Best Practice 6—avoid soiling of laboratory investigation requision slip.

Rationale: Every pathological laboratory item might harboring the potential pathogens. Soiling of requisition slips may act as carrier of infections to ward boys, nursing staff, and other who generally don't use gloves while handling these slips.

Best Practice 7—make hand washing a habit.

Rationale: Hands are most notorious in spreading infection from caregiver to patient or from patient to caregiver. This cross infection ranges from mild to life-threatening infections. Hands can carry infections from one place to another or from one patient to another very rapidly. The practice of hand washing will prevent such cross infections. It is to remember that all 6 steps of hand washing must be followed religiously to make hand safe for patient care.

Best Practice 8—attend training regularly.

Rationale: Training gives updates on the topic and also helps to enhance knowledge, attitude and practice towards assigned training. This way it helps to reduce the incidences of cross infections among staff members. Training may be class room based or on site they are equally effective. Training helps to refresh the practices which are being followed by quite some time. The updates in particular field are shared by trainers to trainees which further increases the safety. "Training activity should be taken as duty not obligation" by staff.

Best Practice 9—read and understand safety protocols.

Rationale: Protocols refresh the memories when they are read and understood. These protocols should be available to all staff members at all places. They can be displayed in the form of posters, computer wallpapers and screensavers. After reading any point in the protocols not understood staff should not hesitate to ask the concerned person or seniors. Organizaiton should encourage practice of personal interaction and Q&A among staff also junior and seniors.

Best Practice 10—periodic health check up of all healthcare workers and waste handlers.

Rationale: This will help to pick up any infection, if at all, at the earliest stage so can be treated efficiently in time. Every organization has time schedule for periodic health check for employees according to their job. One must stick to this schedule and get checked to be assured of infection free.

11. **What should be the contents of the label on container?**
    Date of collection
    Date of generation
    Place of generation
    Waste category
    For off-site/on-site treatment
    Waste handler's name.

12. **Why is labeling of the bag/container important?**
    Because:
    - In case of accident person/staff affected or responsible can be exactly traced.
    - It warns the general public about the hazardous nature of waste.
    - Labeling can be done as hand written or filling of preprinted labels.

13. **How is the BMW transported for off-site storage and treatment?**
    It is transported in bigger vehicle which is having leak proof and corrosive resistant compartments and door having lock facility to secure the waste.

14. **Transport vehicle should have what types of characteristics in it?**
    - Detailed information, i.e. name, address, telephone number of the transporter
    - Body should be leak proof, corrosive resistant and fully enclosed
    - All the corners should be made rounded for easy cleaning
    - There should be no projected part inside the cabin otherwise it will tear the bag

Transport and Storage

- There should be separate cabin for different class of waste
- Vehicle should have enough space so there is no over-crowding of bags
- Vehicle should be designed in such a way that it prevents the discharge of infectious fluid into environment or enroot
- Vehicle should be cleaned thoroughly and disinfected immediately after unload
- Door of vehicle should be close tightly and locked
- Inside should be lined with aluminum.

15. **What details are noted about waste before transport of waste?**
    Following details are noted on consignment note in duplicate of which one cape is given to generator and counter cape is carried by the transporter:
    - Details of name, address and telephone number of waste generator and transporter
    - Name and signature of authorized representative from generator and who is receiving waste
    - Date, type and quantity (category wise) of the waste collection (Fig. 5.2).

Name of the Institution ....

Date ....   **Time** ....

Category of waste	Quantity (kg)	Signature of generator	Signature of collector

Fig. 5.2: Format for waste collection record.

16. **What are the minimum requirement for off-site transportation?**
    - Transport plan and route is approved by the competent authorities

- Waste is transported in leak proof container
- Waste is transported routinely
- Health care facility is aware of final disposal of its waste.

17. **What are the specifications for the route of transportation of internal and/or external waste?**
    - The route for transportation is fixed and logically planned
    - Revised or contingency route plan should also be kept ready in case original plan is not feasible or need alteration
    - Route plan should be practically feasible
    - The collection should starts from the farthest place to nearest place to the storage or treatment area
    - Collection and waste should ideally be start at the beginning of working shift
    - Transport route should be shortest possible route and away from general area.

18. **What is storage of waste?**
    It is the process of storing the waste before it is sent for final treatment/disposal, storage may be in the hospital or outside hospital.

19. **What is the maximum period of untreated waste storage?**
    48 hrs and if this time is to be prolonged then permission from the competent authority is needed.

20. **What are the recommendations for proper storage?**
    - All waste containers should be securely closed and sealed
    - Filled plastic bags are placed in containers and they are also sealed
    - Storage area should be specified and there should be no mixing of the waste.

21. **Mention the recommendations for storage facilities.**
    - Location of the storage area should be big enough to accommodate required number of bags at a time
    - Storage area should have hard cemented flooring with proper drainage facility, so it is easy to clean and disinfect and does not allow any liquid to seep through
    - Waste collection vehicle has easy access to storage area
    - Not accessible to unauthorized person and stray animals
    - Should have double channel door for proper security
    - There should be protection from sun

- Facility should be provided if waste is to be stored for more than 48 hours and in that case area should be earmarked whose temperature does not exceed 10°C
- There should be continuous water supply
- Storage area should have good ventilation and light facilities
- It should be quite far from general water and food storage area of the health care facility
- There should be sufficient supply of protective clothing for the workers
- For on-site treatment facility storage should be in proximity to treatment facility
- Walls and floor of storage area should be free of any crack, gap or breaks
- First aid box should be made available in storage area
- Fire extinguisher should be available in store area
- Separate area should be marked for infectious and non-infectious waste.

22. **What is intermediate storage?**

This is the facility which is available with healthcare facility so as to avoid accumulation and decomposition of waste before it is transported to central facility. In this designated place large containers are placed in which waste is collected. The intermediate storage area should not be accessible to unauthorized persons and have closed containers.

23. **What is centralized storage?**

This is the waste storage are in between intermediate and transportation to external agencies.

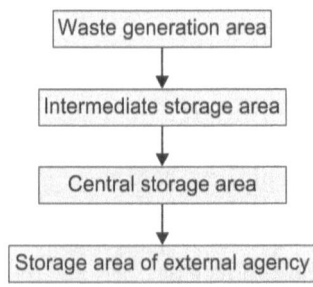

Chapter 6

Treatment and Disposal of Waste

1. **What do you understand by treatment of waste?**
   The process of changing the composition and characteristics of any biomedical waste so as to make it non-infectious and neutral in reaction.

2. **Why there are different methods for biomedical waste treatment/disposal?**
   The physicochemical and biological nature of variety of components in biomedical waste having different magnitude of toxicity and potential hazard necessitate the use of different methods/options for their treatment/disposal.

3. **What should be the prerequisite for choosing treatment method?**
   Method should be:
   - Effective in treating the waste
   - Cost effective
   - Operable
   - Safe for human health and environment.

4. **What is pretreatment?**
   The infectious waste cannot be sent for final disposal without being disinfected first and process of disinfection of waste is called pretreatment.

5. **What are the methods which are used for treatment?**
   - Chemical disinfection
   - Microwave
   - Autoclave
   - Hydroclave.

6. **What are the main methods for treatment of biomedical waste?**
   There are mainly 5 broad categories of treatment methods:
   a. Thermal treatment burn
   b. Mechanical treatment
   c. Chemical treatment
   d. Irradiation treatment
   e. Biological treatment.

7. **Give brief account of various methods of waste treatment.**
   - **Thermal treatment:** This method uses heat in order to decontaminate the waste. Various methods are being used:
     - Incinerator
     - Plasma cytolysis/burn technologies
     - Autoclave
     - Hydroclave/non-burn technologies
     - Microwave.
   - **Mechanical treatment:** Mechanical methods are used to destroy the biomedical waste. These methods used once the waste has been made non-infectious:
     - Granulation
     - Pulping
     - Grinding
     - Compaction
     - Shredding
   - **Chemical treatment:** This method uses chemical disinfectant and mainly used for sharps and plastic wastes. Main solution used are hypochlorite and common bleach.
   - **Irradiation treatment:** Using ionizing radiation the waste is decontaminated. Not much used routinely.
   - **Biological treatment:** This technology uses enzymes for treating medical waste. This method is useful for the waste other than strays, incinerator ash, plastic and human tissues. Methods are:
     - Composting
     - Vermiculture
     - Biodigestion.

8. **Which material is suitable for incinerator?**
   - Human waste
   - Animal waste
   - Laboratory waste

- Contaminated solid waste—like cotton, dressing material, linen, plaster casts, etc.

Category 1, 2, 3, 6 material are directly sent for incineration without chemical pretreatment.

9. **Name the items which should not be incinerated.**
   - Chemical waste
   - Chlorinated plastic waste
   - Pressurized containers
   - Waste with high cadmium and mercury contents
   - Sealed ampules.

10. **What are the characteristics of waste which is suitable for incinerator?**
    - Waste having more than 60% of combustible material
    - Waste having less than 30% of moisture contents
    - Waste having low heating value, i.e. burns at low temperature
    - Waste having less than 5% of non-combustible solids.

11. **What are the types of waste which are not incinerated?**
    - Batteries
    - X-ray or photographic films
    - Mercury thermometers
    - PVC plastics, aerosol cans, gas containers
    - Glass vials which can get melt and block incinerator grate or can explode if uncapped
    - Noncombustible waste.

12. **How the waste with multiple characterstics are treated?**
    During patient care there will be generation of waste which will have multiple characteristics like plastic tubing with cytotoxins or radioactive sharps or urine after radioactive treatment and each characteristic needs separate mode of management hence these waste must be managed with extra caution. In such circumstance the waste must first be treated as hazardous waste and once hazard is removed then recategorized as infectious plastic, glass, sharps, etc. and treated accordingly.

13. **How the waste in white container is treated before final disposal?**
    The waste from white container is treated by autoclaving or dry heat sterilization followed by shredding or mutilation or encapsulation in metal container or cement concrete.

The waste which treated by shredding cum autoclaving is sent for final disposal to iron foundries or sanitary landfill or designated concrete waste sharp pit.

The iron foundries where the metallic sharp is sent for final disposal should have written consent to operate from the State Pollution Control Boards or Pollution Control Committees.

14. **How the waste in blue box is treated?**

    The waste in blue bag/box is treated disinfection (by soaking the washed glass waste after cleaning with detergent and sodium hypochlorite treatment) or through autoclaving or microwaving or hydroclaving and then sent for recycling.

15. **What are the prerequisite for final disposal by deep burial?**
    - The final disposal by deep burial is permitted only in rural or remote areas where common biomedical waste treatment facility cannot reach.
    - The process of deep burial is carried out with prior approval from the prescribed authority.
    - For deep burial the standards are specified in Schedule-III of BMWM rules.
    - The deep burial facility shall be located as per the provisions and guidelines issued by Central Pollution Control Board which are amended from time to time.

16. **What is the specification for chemical treatment?**

    Chemical treatment is used before treatment of waste and should be done by using at least 10% sodium hypochlorite having 30% residual chlorine for 20 minutes or any other equivalent chemical reagent that should demonstrate Log10^4 reduction efficiency for microorganisms as given in Schedule-III of BMWM rules.

17. **What is the purpose of shredding/mutilation of waste?**

    The main purpose is to prevent unauthorized reuse of discarded waste.

18. **How the dead fetus should be managed?**

    As per MTP Act 1971 (amended from time to time) the dead fetus below viability period should be considered as human anatomical waste. This should be collected in yellow bag along with copy of certificate from obstetrician or medical superintendent or head of organization. This official MTP certificate should be prepared in triplicate. One goes to common treatment facility, one remains as official record and one goes to patient file.

19. **What is protocol for management of cytotoxic drug vial?**
    Cytotoxic drug vial can be managed any of the two ways:
    1. Vials should be sent back to manufacturer at single point
    2. Sent to common treatment facility for incineration or plasma pyrolisis (temp > 1200°C)

    A word of caution—vials should not go to any unauthorized person under any circumstance.

20. **How discarded disinfectants/residual chemicals are managed by hospital?**
    Residual or discarded chemicals and used or discarded disinfectants and chemicals should be disposed hazardous waste. This waste should be sent to common treatment facility for further management as per laid down criteria.

21. **Where NACO/WHO guidelines are followed in BMWM?**
    The NACO or WHO guidelines are followed for pretreatment of blood samples, blood bags, laboratory waste and microbiology waste. Once pretreatment is complete then this waste will be sent to common treatment and disposal facility.

22. **What method be used for management of used syringes?**
    Syringes should be mutilated and stored in leak proof container and sent to common facility. In case facility does not have disposal facility then it is the responsibility of hospital to sterilize and dispose as per prescribed and laid down rules.

23. **When biomedical waste is generated at home and how it is managed?**
    In household waste is generated during the caregiving activities like dressing, hence these wastes can be segregated as per rules and handed over to municipal waste collector. The municipality in turn has tie up with common treatment and disposal facility to collect waste from Material recovery facility (MRF) or directly from house to house.

24. **How the waste of red bin is treated and disposed?**
    The waste in red bin is treated by autoclaving or microwaving/hydroclaving followed by shredding or mutilation or combination of sterilization and shredding. Once treated the waste is sent to authorized recyclers or for energy recovery or plastics to diesel or fuel oil or for road making, whichever is possible.

    The organization should take precautions that plastic waste should not be sent to landfill sites in any circumstance.

25. **What is the protocol for management of discarded medicines?**
    All the discarded medicines are managed two ways:
    1. Send them back to dealer/manufacturer
    2. Treated and disposed by incineration

26. **What is the principle of incinerator?**
    By using heat at very high temperature and dry oxidation process it reduces the organic and combustible material into non-combustible and inorganic material reducing the weight and volume of the waste.

27. **What is prerequisite for autoclaving?**
    Prerequisites: Ideally each autoclave should have graphic or computer recording devices which will automatically and continuously monitor and record dates, time of day, load identification number and operating parameters throughout the entire length of the autoclave cycle. All records to be kept for 5 years.

28. **How the validation test of autoclave is done?**
    Use four biological indicator strips, one is used as a control and left at room temperature, three will be placed in the approximate center of three containers with the waste.
    Frequency: Conduct this test three consecutive times to define the minimum operating conditions. The temperature, pressure and residence time at which all biological indicator vials or strips for three consecutive tests show complete inactivation of the spores.
    Follow-on action once in three months and maintain records.

29. **Briefly describe the types of incinerators.**
    - **Single chamber:** Only one chamber with dormancy. This can be mode either with iron drum or bricks. This is the simplest form of incinerator (Fig. 6.1). These incinerator do not have air pollution control device thus cause pollution hence not advocated.
    - **Double chamber incinerators:** Commonly used incinerator. First chamber is called pyrolytic chamber while second chamber is called post-combustion chamber.
    - The temperature in 1st chamber is about 800 (+/−) 50°C and in second chamber 1000 (+/−) 50°C.

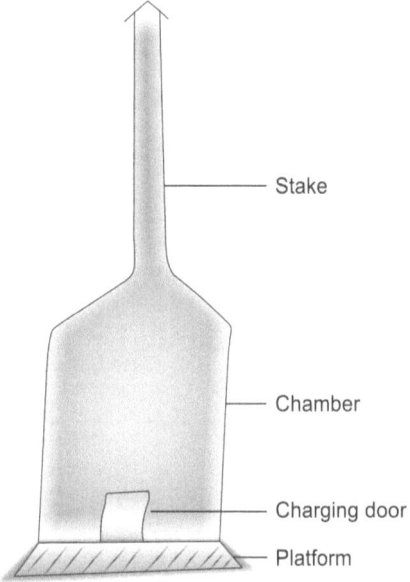

Fig. 6.1: Single chamber incinerator.

- First chamber has less oxygen supply while second chamber has excessive O_2 supply to minimize odor and smoke (Fig. 6.2).
- **Rotary kilns:** It consists of rotating cylindrical chamber lined with fire bricks and a post-combustion chamber. This is specifically used for incinerating chemical waste.

  The rotating oven is inclined at a slight angle and moves 3-5 rotations per minute. The charging of the waste has been done from the top. The residence time in post-combustion chamber is 2 sec.
- **Controlled air incinerator:** In this type of incinerator the O_2 requirement in primary chamber is 40-80% while in secondary chamber 100-150%. In primary chamber the waste is dried, heated and burnt.

30. **What are main pollutants released from incincrators?**
    - Carbon mono-oxide, carbon dioxide and nitrogen oxide.
    - Dioxin and furans
    - Hydrogen chloride
    - Particulate matter
    - Toxic metal fumes.

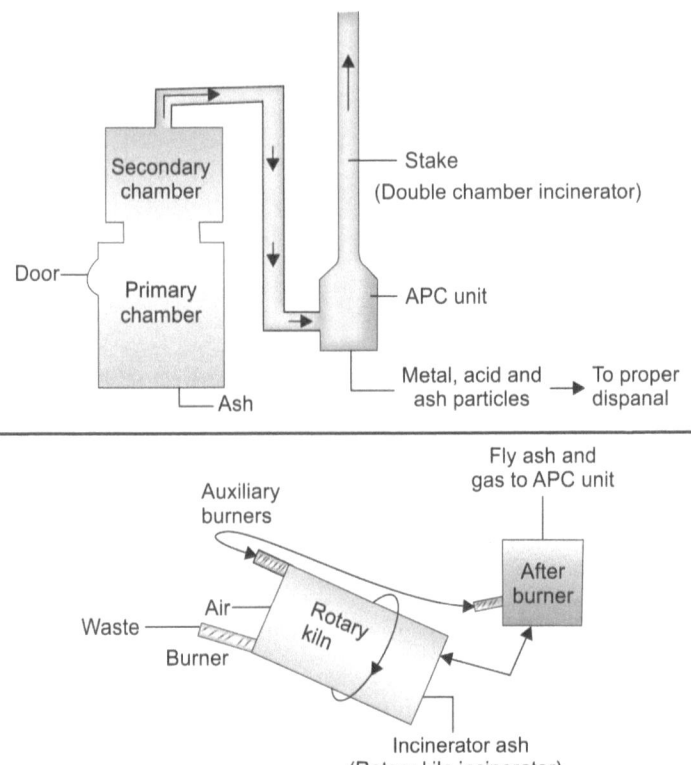

Fig. 6.2: Double chamber incinerator.

31. **Why air pollution control unit be associated with incinerator?**

    Because the chemicals in the waste on burning produce new chemicals which goes into air with emersion and causes air pollution. APC unit does not prevent the formation of pollutants but prevents the release of pollutants into air and get collected either in ash or in air filter.

32. **Name the various types of APC units.**
    - Scrubber (wet and dry)
    - Gravity settler
    - Exhaust fan
    - Dilution equipment
    - Acid gas control, etc.

Treatment and Disposal of Waste

33. What are characteristics of high pressure venturi scrubber?
- Has minimum pressure drop
- Temperature of gas at outlet of scrubber is 70-80°C to ensure saturation of gas
- Made of stainless steel (316 liters) or mild steel lined with acid resistance bricks
- Scrubbing medium circulates at the rate of 2-2.5 liters/m^3 of saturated gas at venturi outlet
- Caustic soda solution is added to venturi system to make medium with pH of around 6.5-7.

34. What are other types of scrubbers system?
- Dry scrubber using lime as filter
- Wet scrubber uses water as filter
- Cyclonic scrubber in which gas circulates in high speed spiral movements with centrifugal force thus particulate matter is separated.
- Centrifugal type droplet separator removes water droplets. The gas/smoke passes through the scrubber.

35. What do you understand by flue (exhaust) gas?
The emission from the incinerator is known as flue gas which contains fly ash.

The flue gas contains heavy metals, water duplets, dioxin furans, carbon dioxide, SO_2, NO_2, H_2S, and particulate matters.

They are treated in two stages:
1. Dedusting—to remove fly ash
2. Washing of gas with alkaline solution—to neutralize oxides of sulfur and halides of hydrogen.

36. How flue gas can be neutralized?
The temperature of flue gas is around 800°C and needs cooling before going for dedusting and the cooling system which is used for flue gas has hot water which can further be used to preheat the waste.

37. Why incinerator ash is disposed carefully?
Because it contains toxins and heavy metals which may produce adverse health and environment effect hence, should be disposed in secured landfill rather than disposing in municipal containers of sewer system.

38. **What is principle of plasma pyrolysis?**
    The principle of plasma pyrolysis is to reduce the material to its basic chemical components by means of very high temperature of gas plasma in the absence of oxygen.

39. **What is plasma arc?**
    It is the thermal treatment system in which the temperature is raised upto 10,000 degrees (Fig. 6.3).

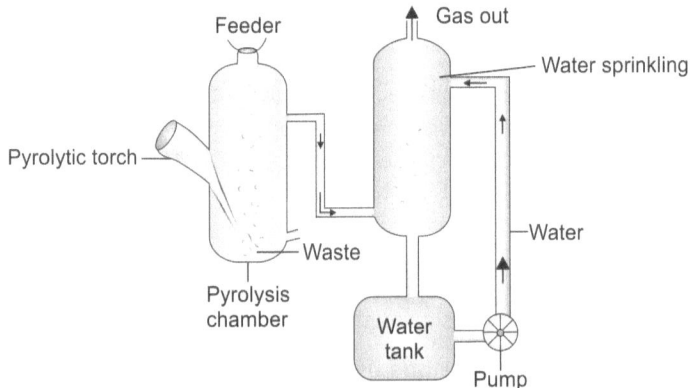

Fig. 6.3: Thermal treatment.

40. **What are advantages of plasma pyrolysis?**
    - Waste is reduced to 1/200th of original volume
    - Waste is reduced to its basic chemical components
    - No furans or dioxin as there is no burning in absence of oxygen
    - It produces a combustible gas as byproduct which can be reutilized
    - Process is not interfered by moisture content of waste.

41. **Mention the disadvantages of plasma pyrolysis?**
    - To produce very high temperature it requires large amount of electrical energy to operate
    - Running cost of system is very high
    - It does produce environment pollution though at lesser degrees.

42. **What is the principle of hydroclave?**
    It works on indirect thermal treatment in which the steam of outer jacket heats up the inner jacket which again produces the steam from the moisture contents of the waste (Fig. 6.4).

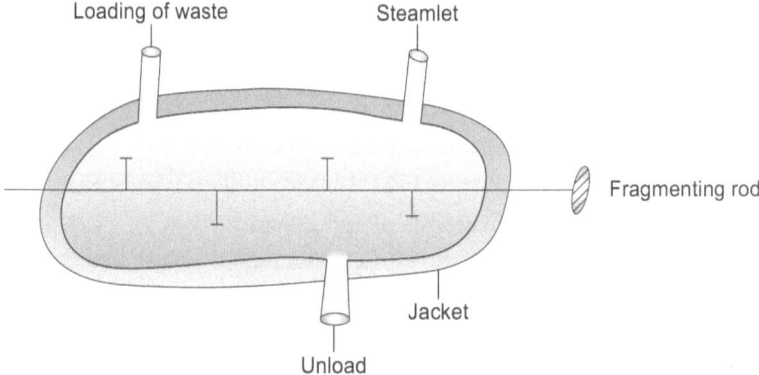

Fig. 6.4: Hydroclave.

43. **What is the main difference between autoclave and hydroclave?**
    In autoclave there is direct contact of steam with the waste while this is not so in hydroclave.

44. **Make the process flowchart of hydroclave.**

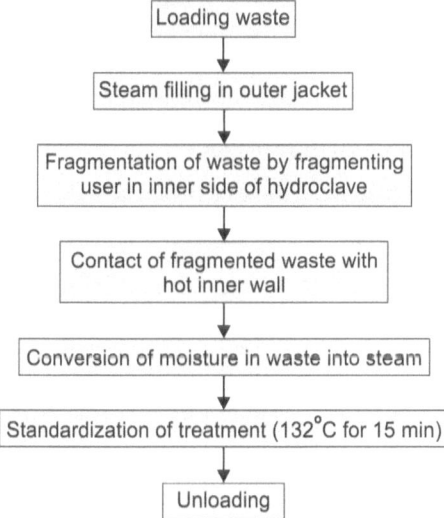

64 Treatment and Disposal of Waste

45. Mention the advantages of hydroclave.
- The waste is reduced in volume as well as in weight by 60-80%
- No hazardous by product as incinerator
- There is no need of waste fragmentation of waste after autoclaving
- Less amount of steam needed to sterilize the waste.

46. Enumerate the disadvantages of hydroclave.
- Not suitable for certain types of waste like chemical, pharmaceuticals and radioactive waste
- Costly installation and operation as compared to autoclave.

47. What is the basic principle of autoclave?
Steam at high temperature and under high pressure inactivates the microorganism then making the waste non-infectious.

48. What are the types of autoclave?
- **Pre-vacuum type autoclave:** Vacuum pump is used to remove the air from treatment chamber then steam is introduced.
- **Gravity type autoclave:** Steam under pressure is used to evacuate the air from chamber.

Pre-vacuum	Gravity type
More efficient	Less efficient
Cycle time 30-60 min.	60-90 min
Operating temp 132°C	120°C

49. What is the process difference between microwave and autoclave?
In autoclave process followed by shredding and microwave shredding followed by process.

50. Mention the step in autoclave process.

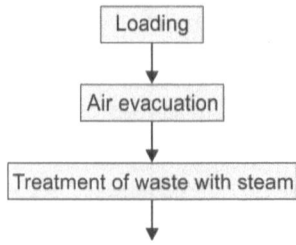

Contd...

Contd...

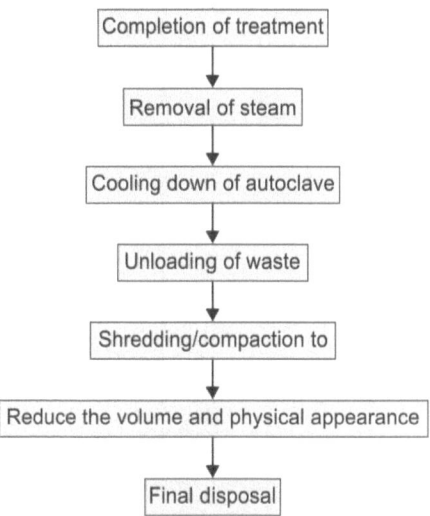

51. **How X-ray waste is disposed off?**
    Developer: Should not be mixed with fixer solution. Developer can be drained into hospital sewer system.
    Fixer: Considered hazardous because high silver contests ionic silver acts as enzyme inhibitor in metabolic process. Fixer is sent to silver recovery system.
    X-ray lead foil/lead shield: Contains pure lead hence sent to recycle system.

52. **What are the advantages of autoclave?**
    - No hazardous byproduct
    - Easy to operate
    - Effective treatment of waste
    - Low capital and operating cost
    - Can be adjusted in small available space as available in different capacities.

53. **What are the disadvantages of autoclave?**
    - Physical appearance not changed hence post-treatment mechanical treatment is needed
    - Fumes emitted have offensive odor
    - Not suitable for cytotoxic, radioactive wastes.

54. What is the working principle of microwave?

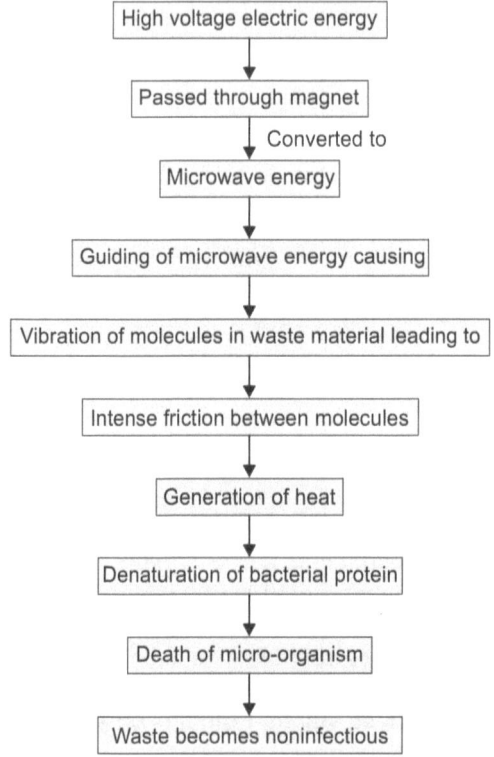

55. What is sterilization by superheated steam?
In this method sterilization of the waste is done with the steam at very high temperature (500 to 700°C) under increased pressure. The shredder is also incorporated with sterilization.

56. What are the advantages of superheated steam sterilization?
- This technology can handle low level radioactive and chlorinated plastic waste
- 50 to 80% reduction in waste achieved.

57. What is wet oxidation technology?
This technology uses oxidation chamber and shredder for the complete treatment of the waste.

The shredded waste is placed in chamber and treated with 10% sulfuric acid and iron ion catalyst where former causes oxidation while the agitation of the chamber ensures treatment of all waste material. The treated waste then placed in rinse chamber where water is sprayed over treated material to remove extra solution.

The technology resembles the washing machine and the method is so rapid that it can treat larger quantity of waste in short time.

58. Write characteristics of microwave.
- They are electromagnetic radiation
- Frequency in between 300-300,000 megahertz.
- Cause heating of material from inside.
- Presence of water intensifies the heating process.

59. What are the advantages of microwave?
- Easy to use
- Due to provision of filters absence of harmful air
- Automatic safe process
- Reduced volume of waste
- Volume of waste reduced significantly
- Absence of liquid discharge.

60. What are the disadvantages?
- High capital cost
- Offensive odor
- May omit toxic contaminants
- Unsuitable for category 1 waste.

61. Mention the methods of treatment in short for sharps, disposable items and liquid waste.
- Broken glass, scraper blades—disinfection with hypochlorite solution
- Needle and syringe nozzel—shredded in needle destroyer and syringe cutter
- Culture plates—autoclave then media disposed off and culture plate reused
- Disposable item—disinfection in freshly prepared 1% sodium hypochlorite solution for 30-60 minutes then shredded before disposal
- Teeth with amalgam—disinfection in glutaraldehyde for 30 min. It should not be sent for incineration because it will lead to emission of mercury in air

Treatment and Disposal of Waste

- Non-infectious liquid waste—neutralized with reagent
- Infectious liquid waste is treated with chemical disinfectant then neutralized.

62. What are the characteristics of treated waste through various methods?

Incinerator	Autoclave	Hydroclave	Microwave	Chemical treatment
Mostly ash and all material unrecognizable. Ash may contain toxic substances	Treated material is wet because of moisture and all material is recognizable	Treated material dehydrated and unrecognizable	Treated waste is wet and later shredded	The waste material which is treated with chemicals is wet in nature and containing traces of chemical which has been used to treat

63. How X-ray fixture solution is managed?

This solution is considered hazardous waste as it contains very high level of silver in it. While in environment free ionic silver acts as enzyme inhibitor thus interfering with metabolic process of organisms. Because of this reason this solution need to be managed either of two ways one is transport it to silver recovery system while second is manage it taking all due precautions for hazardous waste.

64. How cleaner solution is managed?

It is important to note that many of cleaners for developer systems contain chromium which is hazardous material hence treated and managed as hazardous material.

65. How the lead shields/lead foils are managed?

Lead is a heavy metal and in lead, foils and shields are present in pure form. Lead is potentially hazardous to neurological system development and functioning. It can leach from landfills to environment hence managed as hazardous material or lead shields and foils can be sent to metal recovery system.

66. **What is radioactive effluent?**
   The liquid form of radioactive waste is generated from various sources like body imaging, decontamination of radioactive pills, scintillation liquids used in radioimmunoassay (RIA), or chemical or biological research. This liquid form of radioactive waste is known as radioactive effluent.

67. **Describe briefly other treatment methods for waste.**
   Methods in used are:
   - Demolizer
   - KC medical waste technology
   - Electron beam
   - Pyroxidizer
   - Steam reforming.

68. **What are the basic types of chemical treatment methods?**
   - Non-chlorinated: In non-chlorinated methods glutaraldehyde, peracetic acid or ozone is used.
   - Chlorinated: In chlorinated method sodium hypochlorite is mainly used.

69. **What are the suitable articles for chemical disinfection?**
   - Plastic
   - Rubber
   - Metallic item.

70. **What is the prerequisite for chemical disinfections?**
   Shredding of the waste material is the prerequisite for chemical disinfection. It has following purpose:
   - Shredding reduces the volume of waste
   - It increases the surface area for action of chemicals
   - Shredding eliminates the closed space of waste item.

71. **What is the recommended dilution of sodium hypochlorite for blood spill treatment?**
   100 ml/liter with 1% available chlorine (10 gm/ltr = 10,000 ppm).

72. **What is the contact period for different chemical agents?**
   Household bleach contains 4-5% of available chlorine. However, it can be utilized after diluting to have 1% available chlorine. The minimum contact period is 30 minutes.

73. **What are other chemical disinfectants effective in activating HIV?**

70% ethanol	3-5 min
2% povidone iodine	15 min
2% glutaraldehyde (cidex)	30 min
6% hydrogen peroxide	30 min
4% formaline	30 min.

74. **How sodium hypochlorite is formed?**

    $2Cl_2 + 2NaOH + H_2O \rightarrow 2NaOCl$ (sodium hypochlorite) $+ 2HCl$

75. **Which waste is unsuitable for chemical treatment?**
    - Cytotoxic agents
    - Volatile and semivolatile organic compounds
    - Mercury
    - Radiological waste.

76. **What are the advantages of chemical treatment?**
    - Liquid effluent can be safely discharged into sewer system
    - Waste unrecognizable
    - No byproduct.

77. **What are the disadvantages of clinical treatment?**
    - Chemical itself is hazardous
    - Ineffective for large quantity of waste at a time.

78. **Why radiations are not used for waste treatment?**
    - Because there is no change in volume, weight and shape of the waste
    - Y radiations are ionizing radiation extremely harmful
    - Not suitable for category 1 and chemical waste.

79. **What precautions should be taken while handling and storing chemical?**
    - Proper labeling of the chemical containers
    - Prompt identifications of chemical hazard
    - Standard operating procedure (SOP) for chemical safety
    - Workers training to reduce hazards from chemicals
    - Replacement of chlorinated solvents by less hazardous chemicals
    - Unused/expired chemical to be returned to supplier as mentioned in contract

- Proper record-keeping of all chemicals
- Record keeping of chemical exposures and immediate management of such exposure
- Use of personal protective measures.

80. **Which biological methods are used for hospital waste?**
    - Biodigestion
    - Vermiculture
    - Pit composting

    These are suitable for rural health institutions.

81. **Which type of waste is suitable for biological methods?**

    Waste which is not infectious is suitable for biological treatment and disposal. Hospital kitchen waste, leftover food, fruit peels, vegetables, etc.

82. **Briefly describe the biological process (Fig. 6.5).**
    - **Biodigestion:** Also called aerobic digestion. This is similar to biogas system. However, instead of gobar other waste like kitchen waste, leftover food is used. The process is fed daily and equal quantity of slurry is formed which is released into slurry pit where manure is formed. Cow dung may be used as initial biodigester. In the process methane gas is formed which is collected at the dome of the system and is ready for being used as cooking fuel. This method is suitable for rural area institution where considerable noninfectious waste is produced.
    - **Vermiculture:** This is another ecofriendly treatment and disposal method suitable for biodegradable waste.

      In this method cow dung, coconut husk and earthworms (Eisenia fetida) are used.

      Dimensions of pit: 3 feet wide and 8-10 inches deep made of wooden box of the same size used.

      Layers in pit
      – First layer rubber to prevent worm from escaping
         Second layer coconut husk to retain moisture.
      – Third layer cowdung about 6 inches in height.
      – Fourth layer earthworm half the weight of cow dung.

      Mature: Pit should be watered daily for few days. Then divide the pit in 7 segments and one segment is used for a day and at the end of week first week is refed, while keeping the pit moist.

After 6 weeks: Remove the manure and put them in direct sunlight and reuse the pit.
Precautions: Avoid putting plastic or metal waste in pit.
- **Pit composing:** Here instead of earthworm cowdung is used for treating and disposing biodegradable waste.

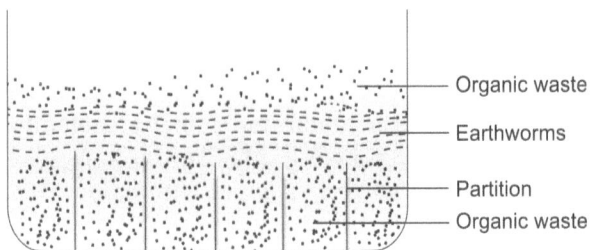

Fig. 6.5: Vermiculture box.

83. **On what factors the efficiency of chemical disinfectants depend?**
    - Type of chemical
    - Contact time
    - Amount of chemical used
    - Operating temperature, pH
    - Organic load of the waste.

84. **What factors are considered before a chemical disinfectant is chosen for the use?**
    - Cost
    - Effectivity
    - Duration of effectivity
    - Post use disposal.

85. **What are the commonly used disposal methods?**
    - Deep burial
    - Sanitary land fills
    - Encapsulation
    - Shredding.

86. **Explain in brief the disposal methods of waste.**
    - **Deep burial:** It is a small pit which is secured by high barbed wire fence. The pit is usually 1-2 meters in diameter and 2-5

meters depth. The waste is disposed in pit and covers with soil or soil plus lime of 10-20 cm thick layer. When the pit is filled about 50 cm from the brain it is covered with a layer of cement or wire wash over which soil is filled which gives about 50 cm cover. On the basis of pit earth wound are made to prevent water entering into pit (Fig. 6.6).

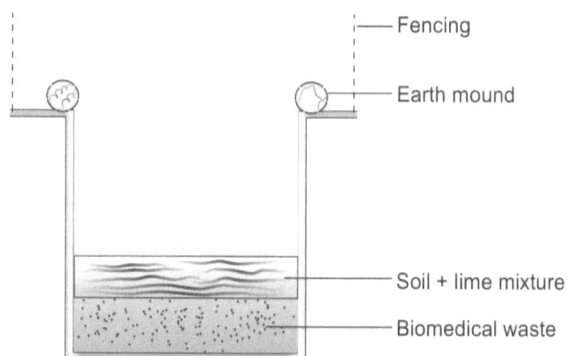

Fig. 6.6: Deep burial pit.

- **Sanitary landfills:** There are landfills with advanced engineering complexity. These have following central measures:
    - Gas control
    - Environmental monitoring points
    - Bore holes for monitoring round water and air quality.

  This needs following specialized components:
    - Trained workforce
    - Security of the landfill area
    - Overhead cover to prevent rain water retaining into it
    - License for using the place
    - Site away from residential area
    - Easy approach for transport vehicle
    - Depth of landfill should be around 2 meters to avoid scavenging and accidental recovery of waste
    - Pit should be at least 100 meters away from ground water source
    - Should not be located near the flood prone area.

87. **What are the types of needle destroyers?**
    - **Mechanical:** In mechanical type needle destroyer the needle is sheared from the syringe with the help of lever and collected in box.
    - **Electrically operated:** In electrically operated needle destroyer the needle is either sheared or destroyed by platinum plate leaving a residue of steel at heated around 700–800°C. In both the types only one needle can be sheared at a time along with this the leaver is also able to destroy the tip of syringe to make it unusable.

88. **What is encapsulation?**
    This is the process of mixing the waste with encapsulating material to make the whole material hard and unusable. This can be done either in drum on ground pit. This is mainly used for sharp waste (Fig. 6.7).

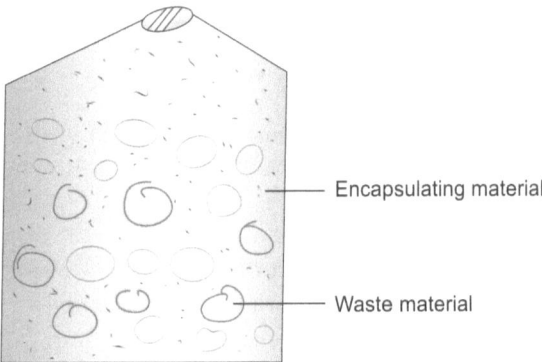

Fig. 6.7: Encapsulation.

89. **What are the encapsulating materials used?**
    - Cement
    - Clay
    - Bituminous sand, etc.

90. **What is shredder?**
    Shredder is a machine which is used to make waste unrecognizable after treatment. This is mainly used for plastic waste which after shredding can be recycled.

This can be either multiple shaft or single shaft shredder. It has automatic safety device which shuts off the machine in case the operation is not correct to avoid any accident.

91. **What is the composition of encapsulation material?**
    1 part cement
    1 part lime
    4 parts sand
    ½ part water

92. **What precautions should be taken after needles are mutilated?**
    They should be disinfected in 0.5% hypochlorite solution with contract period of around 30 min. This should strictly be done at the point of waste generation.

93. **Why chlorine compound be used for chemical disinfection?**
    Because they are:
    - Very effective
    - Easy available at cheaper prize
    - Easy to use.

94. **What are demerits of chemical disinfectants?**
    - Not effective against spores
    - Loses effectiveness if chlorine content is lost
    - Need fresh preparation.

95. **Why sharp injury in more important?**
    Because sharp causes dual injuries, one transmission of infection by inoculation and it also causes physical injury.

96. **What are the objectives of sharp injury surveillance program.**
    - The sharp injury surveillance program has two main objectives namely:
        1. Development of more effective safety measures.
        2. Better educational strategies.
    - Healthcare organization should ensure that more and more employees participate in these program.

97. **What should be the main quality of sharp container?**
    - It should be puncture proof to avoid sharp injury
    - Its mouth should be narrow so that sharp cannot be accidentally recovered.

Treatment and Disposal of Waste

98. **How sharps are finally disposed?**

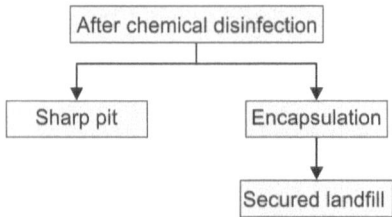

99. **What are the characteristics of sharp pit?**
    - It has cemented walls and floor (Fig. 6.8)
    - It is covered with thick iron or cement slab having circular in which 6 inch diameter pipe is fitted with lid and lock facility
    - Size of pit depends on the waste generation and space availability
    - Once it is filled around 1 foot below cover, then cement slurry is used to fill the pit and next one is prepared.

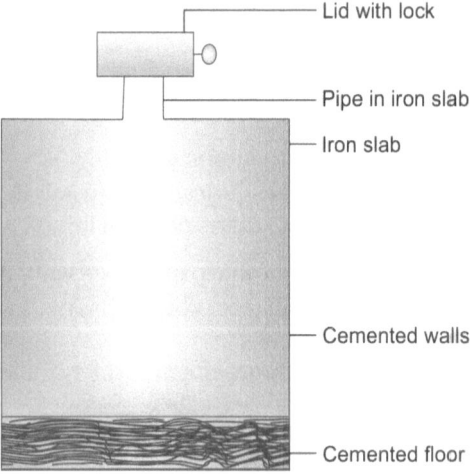

Fig. 6.8: Safe pit for sharps.

100. **How the plastic syringes can be disinfected at the point of generation?**

    This can be done by using two baskets—outer rigid and inner perforated in between hypochlorite solution is filled and syringes are put into inner side which came in contact with disinfectant after contact period of 30 minutes then the bin can be emptied in larger one (Fig. 6.9).

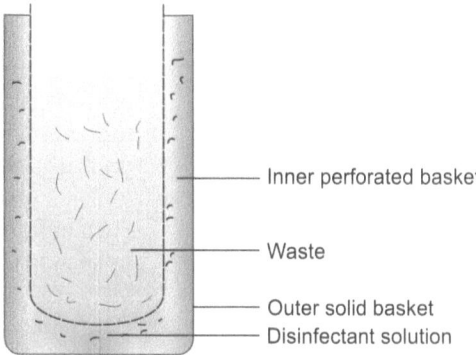

Fig. 6.9: Two-basket system.

101. **Which methods are commonly used for disposal of liquids?**
 - Soak pit
 - Sewers
 - Waste stabilizing plant having aerobic filter and activated sludge technology.

102. **What is average frequency and average length of microwave?**
 Frequency   2450 mHz
 Wavelength   12.24 cm

103. **How is 1% hypochlorite solution prepared?**
 By dissolving 10 gm of bleaching powder in 1 liter of water. The solution has to be prepared fresh every time and changed every 12 hrs.

104. **What are the disposal options for treated medical waste?**
 - Treated solid waste—Municipal landfill
 - Encapsulated sharps—Municipal landfills
 - Disinfected and shredded—Municipal landfills or recycling
 - Incineration ash—Secured landfill
 - Oil and grease—Incineration.

105. **How the sharps and plastic should be treated before shredding?**
 They should be treated by:
 - Chemical disinfectants
 - Microwaving
 - Autoclaving.

106. What is working pattern of microwave system?

Shredding of material → Pushing of material into treatment chamber → Moistening of waste with high temp steam
↓
Microwaving at 95–100°C for residence time 30 min and cycle time around 50 min.
↓
Further fragmentation by second shredder
↓
Discharge of waste into container for landfill.

Chapter 7

Education and Training

1. **What is training?**
   It is the systemic way of giving an information to person about a process or skills.

2. **Which type of training is given in case of biomedical waste management (BMWM)?**
   The training is given based on andragogical model.

3. **Why there is need for proper management of biomedical waste (BMW)?**
   Though a very small portion of total BMW is infectious and hazardous yet to minimize even that percentage in population and for environmental safety the need for proper BMW management arise:
   - Chances of hospital acquired infection because of improper waste management.
   - Sharp injuries which directly inoculating microorganisms in bloodstream of staff and waste handlers thus leading to infections.
   - Disposable items being repacked and sold in the market by unscrupulous elements.
   - Risk of water, air and land pollution due to dumping of untreated waste and incomplete incineration.
   - Risk associated with hazardous chemicals and/or drugs to persons handling these chemicals and waste at all levels in the healthcare organization.
   - Waste medicines are repacked and sold to unsuspecting buyers.
   - Untreated waste dumped may pose risk to general population living in vicinity of such dumping areas.

4. **What should be emphasised during the employee training program on BMWM?**

   Employee training programs on BMWM should cantered around following:
   - Personal hygiene, especially handwashing practices as per policy of organization.
   - Facility's procedures for the reduction, segregation, collection, color coding, labelling, storage, and in-house movement of waste.
   - Prevention methods for transmission of infections waste handling.
   - Chemical exposure hazards which may occur during handling of these chemicals.
   - Awareness about the intimation channels available in organization in case of any incident.

5. **What are the assumptions of adult training model?**
   - Adults have need to know the reason for learning
   - Adults are free to determine what, when and how they should learn
   - Adults are self-directed learners
   - Adults have very sharp sense of understanding
   - Adults learn more in non-formal and unorganized and loosely structured programs.

6. **Which are the target groups for training?**
   - Doctors
   - Nurses
   - Patients' attendants
   - Paramedical staff
   - Waste handlers.

7. **Why do waste handlers need training?**

   Because:
   - They may be in any service bracket
   - They may be from any educational background
   - They are less motivated
   - They are less aware of gravity of hazards posed by BMWM
   - Belong to low socioeconomic groups
   - Sometimes they may bypass the precautionary measures
   - They usually take the instructions lightly.

8. **What are the objectives of training and education?**
   - To make HCW aware of hazards related to BMWM and its indiscriminate handling
   - To prevent the exposure to BMWM
   - To highlight the various stages of BMWM and their importance
   - To initiate better waste handling practices.

9. **How the structured training program is prepared?**
   It can be prepared on weekly or monthly basis. Organization may have policy to impart training for minimum hours of training in a year and include employee's training participation in performance appraisal.

Date	Chapter	Trainer	Time	Venue	Target employee

10. **Which type of teaching is appropriate for waste handlers?**
    Teacher – student – content centered

11. **What methodology is useful for training?**
    - Group discussion
    - Problem solving situation
    - Lectures
    - Modular training
    - Field visits.

12. **On what factor the methodology depends?**
    - Contents of the case
    - Proficiency of trainer
    - Motivation level of learner
    - Type of training to be imparted.

13. **What should be main characteristics of training program?**
    It should be:
    - Consistent

- Universal
- Applied carefully based on evaluation reports
- Periodic evaluation
- Modification of future response.

14. **What training aids are useful?**
    - Posters
        - Booklets
        - Manuals
        - Flip chart
    - OH
        - Video films
    - Practical demonstration
        - Hands on training.

15. **What are the characteristics of andragogy?**
    - Adults are self-directed and show need for training due to inner motivation
    - Adults expect the respect from trainer
    - They have precious experience and knowledge as well
    - Adults are practical in their approach
    - They are result oriented.

16. **What are the qualities of good trainer?**
    - Has good communication skills
    - Able to coordinate with trainee through constructive approach
    - Should be well versed with area of specialization and should be able to identify the gaps
    - Should be willing participant in training program
    - Should keep on updating knowledge, techniques and new methodologies
    - Should be able to get regular feedback from trainees and modify training approach accordingly.

17. **What are the characteristics of good trainees?**
    - Regular for training program
    - Give in time proper feedback to trainer
    - Ask questions to clear doubts
    - Remain attentive during training session
    - Show cooperation and coordination with fellow trainees
    - Actively participate in training program.

18. **What are the characteristics of effective communication?**
    - Proper preparation of subject and training materials
    - Understanding needs of trainees
    - Ensure that trainees are listening and understanding the subject
    - Does not use too much of technical language
    - Quickly establishes good interpersonal relations with trainees
    - Trainer should make trainee listen actively.

19. **What are the possible gaps in BMWM?**
    - Knowledge, skill, and attitude (KSA) gap
    - Technology gap
    - Policy and procedures gap
    - Effective supervisory gap.

20. **What is evaluation of training?**
    It is a process of collecting information which can be utilized for decision-making about present and future training activities.

21. **What are basic questions arise while doing evaluation?**
    - Why to do evaluation?
    - When to do evaluation?
    - What to evaluate?
    - How to evaluate?

22. **What are the basic principles of evaluation?**
    - Clarity of purpose
    - Reliability of results
    - Tailor made evaluation tools
    - Objectivity of evaluation
    - Evaluation is a process not the end product of training
    - Feasibility.

23. **What are the basic qualities of evaluator?**
    - Committed to the process
    - Good interpersonal relationship
    - Helps to realize benefits of training
    - Encourages others to get evaluated.

24. **What are different evaluation methods?**
    Pre-training:
    - Training need identification (TNI)
    - Evaluation of training objectives

- Evaluation of performance standard
- Evaluation of trainees profile.

Post-training:
- Reaction evaluation
- Learning evaluation
- Job behavior evaluation.

25. **What measures should be taken while giving training to waste handlers?**
    - Training should be given in local language
    - Highlights the importance of proper management
    - Brief account of infectious waste and diseases caused by them
    - Brief introduction of biomedical waste management rules
    - How to cope with accident/injuries?
    - How to maintain personal hygiene?
    - Appreciation to those who follow instructions and punishment for dereliction of duty and noncompliance.

26. **What is capacity building?**
    It consists of various activities which strengthen the knowledge, skill, ability, and behavior of individual in order to achieve organizational goals.

27. **Who all need training in BMW management?**
    Training modules need to be developed for:
    - Medical and laboratory staff
    - Paramedical staff (nurses, ward boys)
    - Housekeeping and security staff (sweepers, cleaners, guards)
    - Administrative staff.

28. **Is contents of training different for different categories?**
    Yes, each category needs different type and content training because of different types involvement and different responsibilities in waste management and for this they need to know:
    - Their specific role regarding BMW management
    - How important is to comply with rules, regulations and policy decisions taken by management of the healthcare facility?
    - Level of their contribution to make BMW management plan successful in the organization.

29. **What should be the content of training module for medical and laboratory staff?**
   The training sessions are conducted as formalized by the head of the institution and during training session detailed discussion between trainer and trainees takes place on:
   - Existing rules and regulations related to BMW management and handling.
   - Hazards and impact of improper waste management on health of the staff and community.
   - Policy of the specific healthcare establishment regarding management of BMW.
   - Step by step management of waste and description of tools and methods involved in each step.
   - Adverse events while handling and managing waste and what measures to be taken to have corrective as well as preventive actions.
   - Role of each staff category in successful management of waste without any adverse event.
   - Feedback from trainee which will be considered subsequently for further betterment of management of waste.

30. **How the feedback is taken from trainees?**
   It should always be taken on the prescribed format in two languages, one local and another English.

31. **What is the format for obtaining feedback?**
   It is given below:

Feedback form for the training Topic .... Date .... Trainer					
Training contents	Excellent	Very good	Good	Satisfactory	Not satisfactory
Text related to training topic					
Training methodology relevant to type of trainees					
Training materials					

Contd...

Contd...

Training contents	Excellent	Very good	Good	Satisfactory	Not satisfactory
Language of training					
Overall impression					

32. **What should be the training module contents for paramedical staff?**

    The training module contents for paramedical staff contains:
    - Impact of improper waste management on staff and population's health
    - Knowledge about existing rules, regulations and policies related to BMW management
    - Knowledge about each step in BMW management process and importance of each step
    - During training session supply of relevant chart depicting practical implications of rules related to BMW management
    - Knowledge about do and don't about BMW
    - Process of adverse incidence reporting
    - Rewards and punishments
    - Case study examples narrating processes and incidences
    - Onsite practicum so that the staff understands more logically
    - Active feedback and consideration of these feedback for betterment of management of waste.

33. **What should be the training module contents for waste handlers, cleaners and security guards staff?**

    Because of their education background and unawareness towards the health hazards the training preferable be done in local language which most understandable to them. The training contents should stress up on.
    - Health hazards of BMW and impact on health by improper management of this waste
    - Brief introduction rules, regulations and organization's policy regarding BMW management
    - Simple method to deliver their responsibilities and how to remain vigilant towards improper waste management

- Maintenance of personal hygiene and proper use of PPE while handling of waste
- Reward and punishment
- Adverse events related to BMW management and how to report to authorities
- Immediate actions to be taken in case of adverse event.

34. **What should be the training module contents for healthcare facility's administrative staff?**

    This capsule would contain material for awareness generation, responsibilities and accountabilities formulation of policy.
    - Awareness generation, highlighting the social, ethical and legal responsibilities of the management, case studies.
    - Discussion on the biomedical waste (Management and Handling) Rules, 1998, its amendments emphasising the legal, financial and contractual issues.
    - The steps required for formulating a policy for the specific healthcare establishment, keeping in view the Govt rules.
    - Co-ordination with the civic and health authorities as well as with the prescribed authority of the State.
    - Administrative and managerial support mechanism necessary for implementing and sustaining a proper biomedical waste management system.
    - How to motivate and elicit co-operation from various staff members.
    - The concept of common treatment facility—legal, financial and contractual issues.

35. **What would be appropriate methods for education on BMWM for general population?**

    The following methods can be considered for public education:
    - Poster exhibitions of healthcare waste issues including risks involved in scavenging discarded syringes and hypodermic needles.
    - Friendly explanation by the hospital staff to all incoming patients, family members and visitors on hospital's waste management policy.
    - Distribution of leafets should be considered to all patients, family members and visitors on hospital's waste management policy.

- Information poster exhibitions throughout the hospitals, at strategic locations, such as waste bin locations giving instructions on waste segregation.
- Posters should exhibit diagrams and illustrations to convey the message as loud and clear as possible, including illiterate people visiting hospital.
- All information should be displayed or communicated in an attractive manner that will hold people's attention.

36. **What will be hospital staff categories who will need training and education on BMWM?**
    - Nurses and assistant nurses
    - Cleaners, porters, auxiliary staff, and waste handlers
    - Medical doctors
    - Hospital managers and administrative staff responsible for implementing regulations on healthcare waste management.

37. **What should be the contents of training and education for hospital staff on BMWM as per policy?**

    The staff training and education program should include the following:
    - Information on, and justification for all aspects of the healthcare waste policy being followed in organization.
    - Information on the role and responsibilities of each hospital staff member in implementing the policy.
    - Technical instructions, relevant for the target group of staff, on the application of waste management practices.
    - Hands-on training of small groups of personnel.
    - Post-training evaluation of all participants using simple MCQ questions.

38. **Is refresher training on BMWM is necessary?**

    Yes. In fact hospital management should make it mandatory to have refreshing training schedule for staff on periodic interval for following reason:
    - Periodic repetition of training will have a chance to provide refreshment and orientation training for new joinees and will confer new responsibilities for existing employees.
    - Repetition in training will update knowledge of the staff in line with policy changes which takes place in every organization

from time to time depending upon new requirement or changes in government policies.
- Follow-up training give an overview to trainers that how much information has been retained by participants and this will guide them about future need of refresher courses.

39. **Who should be made responsible for conducting and monitoring training schedule?**

    The infection control officer (ICO) should be given responsibility for all training related to all stages of biomedical waste management. He/she should ensure that staff at all levels are aware both of the hospital waste management plan and policy and of their own responsibilities and obligations in this regard.

    Infection control officer should be in-charge of keeping all the records related to training sessions, The content of training programs should be periodically reviewed and updated by ICO.

    For similar training of those concerned with smaller sources of healthcare waste, the regional health authority may be able to make centralized arrangements for courses.

    The training package should be liberally illustrated with drawings, diagrams, photographs, slides, or overhead transparencies to make more acceptable by participants and leave long lasting educational effects.

40. **How infection control officer should select participatnts for training?**

    The ideal number of participants in a training course is 20-30 because large groups make effective discussions and exercises difficult to monitor. Training activities should be aimed at all categories of staff members because discussions among diverse group is easier and more useful. It is advisable to include senior administration staff and heads of departments in certain training sessions so as to demonstrate their commitment to the waste management policy and to show the relevance of the policy to all personnel of healthcare organization.

41. **What precautions should be taken for waste generating staff?**
    - While removing needle from syringe the greatest care should be taken.

- In no. of cases items should be remove from waste bin or bag, waste filled bag should never be staked one over another or into another bag.
- Differ colored bags should never be carried togather by staking one over another.
- Hazardous and general waste should not be mixed. If at all by mistake two are mixed, the entire mixture should be treated as hazardous waste.
- Nursing and clinical staff should ensure that adequate numbers of containers are provided for the collection, and subsequent on-site storage.

42. **Mention the salient points to be considered during training of biomedical waste handlers.**
    - Check that waste storage bags and containers are sealed. All bags should be properly labeled and securely sealed before removing from waste bins to prevent spillages.
    - Bags should be picked up by the neck only. They should be put down in such a way that they can again be picked up by holding the neck for further handling.
    - Manual handling of waste bags should be minimized whenever possible.
    - Waste bags should be handled in such a way that it does not touch the body during its movement.
    - Waste collectors should not attempt to carry too many bags at one time—probably not more than two.
    - When process of moving of waste bags or containers is complete, then waste handler should check seal again to ensure that it is intact.
    - To avoid puncture or other damage, waste bags should not be thrown or dropped in trolley or floor.
    - Sharps may occasionally puncture the side or bottom of container hence these containers should never be supported from bottom with another hand.
    - Bags for general and hazardous waste should not be mixed and be placed only in specified storage areas.
    - Appropriate cleaning and disinfection procedures should be followed in the event of accidental spillage and incident should be reported immediately to concerned staff.
    - Adequate personal protective equipment (PPE) should be worn during all waste handling operations.

43. **What should be the points of concerns for training for waste transport staff?**

Drivers and waste handlers who are responsible for transportation of waste from healthcare facility to common treatment facility should be aware of the nature and risks of the transported waste. Ideally transport staff should be trained in the procedures listed below. They should be able to carry out all procedures in accordance with the instructions, without help from others.

- Staff should be knowing correct procedures for handling, loading, and unloading waste bags/containers.
- How to deal with spillages or other occupational accidents. Written standard operating procedures (SOPs) for relevant procedures should be available in the transport vehicle.
- The wearing of PPE should be made mandatory at all times.
- Listed items should be made available in transport vehicle all the time and these items are—plastic bags, PPE, cleaning tools and disinfectants in order to deal with any spillage which may occurs during process of loading, transport, or unloading.
- Documentation and recording of healthcare waste, e.g. by means of a consignment note system. This will help to trace the point of origin of waste.
- Designated staff from healthcare facility should liaise with the transport contractor to ensure that members of the waste collection crew are well-trained. Untrained personnel should never be allowed to handle hazardous healthcare waste.

44. **Write down training points for treatment plant operators.**

Treatment plant operators should have received technical education to at least secondary school level, and should be specifically trained in the following areas:

- General functioning of the treatment facility.
- Health, safety, and environmental implications of treatment operations.
- Technical procedures for operation of the plant.
- Emergency response, in case of equipment failures alarms.
- Surveillance of the quality of ash and emissions, according to the specifications.
- Maintenance of the plant and record-keeping.

45. **Write down the issues to be addressed during training of treatment plant operators.**

Waste handling
- Procedures for receiving, handling, and storage of healthcare waste.
- Loading of waste into the treatment unit.

Operation of the plant
- Operation of the plant equipment including startup and shutdown procedures.
- Operation and testing of control, alarm, and instrumentation systems; corrections where necessary.
- Optimum operating temperatures, pressures, concentrations of emissions, speeds, flows, etc. and maintenance of correct conditions.
- Detection of defects or malfunctions (following SOPs) and servicing.
- Safe removal of residues and ashes.

Maintenance
- Daily, weekly, monthly, semi-annual, and annual tests, inspection, cleaning, lubrication, replacement and replenishment of consumables (e.g. thermocouples), and overhaul with special attention to major components of the installation; appropriate action when necessary.

Safety measures and emergency response
- Use of PPE and personal hygiene.
- Fire precautions.
- Procedures for emergency response including manual operation of the plant under emergency conditions; dealing with spillages, accidents, and other incidents.
- Contingency plans for implementation during breakdown or planned maintenance.

Administrative procedures
- License conditions and regulations governing emissions.
- Record-keeping.
- Reporting of spillages, accidents, and other incidents to concerned authorities.

Chapter 8

Managerial Issues in Biomedical Waste Management

1. **Why hospitals are different from other industries?**
   In every hospital energy and water consumption is very high, production of chemical and nonchemical waste amount is too much, magnitude of potentially dangerous substance output is high, and purchase of consumable materials is tend to be chaotic. Therefore, it is of paramount importance that all departments successfully perform the supply activities in order to provide an effective and fruitful health service outcome. These are the basic reasons which make hospitals different from other industries.

2. **What is green management in hospitals?**
   Green management is a new approach for environment management system and aims to make society to which they render service with activities supporting health and healthy life sustainable. Green management being new approach for environment management system, is a process that comprise reformation aimed at environmental health. The first step is to prevent the environmental pollution at every level and the second step is to provide savings in all kinds of sourcing and tend towards the renewable sources.

   It can be said that green management involves purchase of materials which are recyclable, reusable or that have just been recycled. The process also involves choosing the supplier conforming with the environmental aims, providing savings in using all types of sources, supplying products that make sourcing fruitful. The institute participates by:
   - Using materials, equipments and devices which do not contain hazardous material.

- Reducing the waste materials
- Creating reuse or recycle opportunities
- Making environmental planning
- Developing activities that improve environmentalist perspective thus creating ecological value.

3. **What are key elements of green hospital given by WHO?**

   World health organizations (WHO): has given seven key elements for green hospital and these are as under—
   1. With efficiency measures, reducing cost and energy consumption
   2. Building to reduce resource and energy demand and being sensitive to climate conditions
   3. Producing/consuming clean, renewable energy
   4. Make personnel and people coming to the hospital prefer walking and cycling
   5. Sustainability of producing/consuming green food for personnel and patients
   6. Reducing waste and using alternative disposal techniques
   7. Finding safe alternatives to save water instead of bottled ones.

4. **What is Triple bottom line (TBL/3BL) principle?**

   The triple bottom line is an accounting framework having three components or dimentions: Social, environmental (ecological) and economical (financial). The green supply chain shows concerns regarding environmental and economic performance of

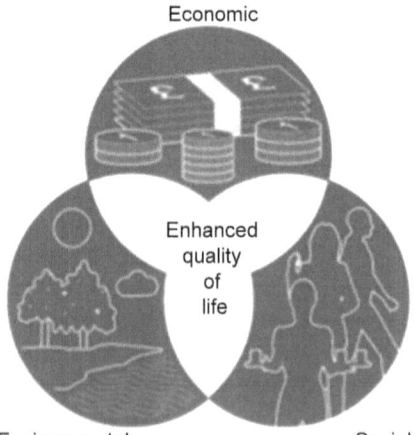

Managerial Issues in Biomedical Waste Management

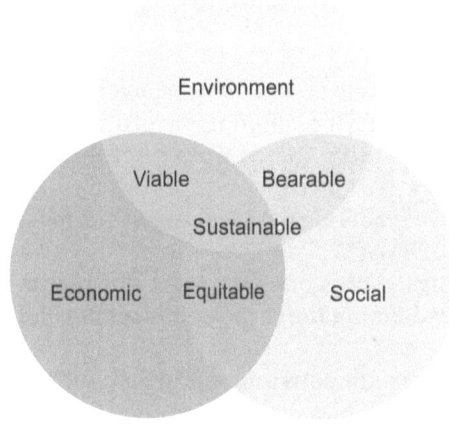

a supply chain. Sustainable supply chain, in its conceptualization, incorporates social dimension as well. This concept intends to address all the dimensions of TBL. Some organizations have adopted the TBL framework to evaluate their performance in a broader perspective to create greater business value.

5. **Why hospitals are in front line for ideal waste management practices?**

    Hospitals and healthcare organizations represent an essential societal function having a fundamental mission to care for and heal the sick. In many respects, healthcare institutions are held to a higher ethical standard than virtually any other enterprise, as to do good, not merely to do well.

6. **What is the role of hospital manager in biomedical waste management (BMWM)?**

    Hospital manager should ensure that biomedical waste is managed in environmentally safe manner.

7. **What are the prerequisites for safe BMWM?**
    - Hospital should have BMWM committee
    - Hospital should develop the policy approved by committee
    - Committee should involve everyone in the hospital in the process
    - Policy and procedures should be received periodically
    - Committee should also evolve the strategy for waste management.

8. **Why should there be strategy?**
   To ensure that all the regulatory requirement related to BMWM are fulfilled.

9. **What are the basic components of an effective strategy?**
   - Clear out living the commitment of the hospital management
   - Clearly defining the commitment towards allocation of resources
   - Precisely rendering the accountability and responsibilities in terms of BMWM
   - Defining the categories of waste being produced
   - Clearly defining the disposal procedures for each category of waste
   - Ensuring continuous training and education.

10. **What is waste audit?**
    It is a valuable tool which helps to understand the type and quantity of waste and involves data collection, analysis, and recommendations. Data can be analyzed manually or through computer software. It is the methodical process of characterizing, quantifying and delineating different waste streams through the waste survey to evolve the waste management policies.

    During audit following information are collected—quantity of waste, type of waste, states of equipment/machines, condition of protective personal clothing, incidence of sharp injuries, disinfection process and spill management process.

11. **What is the main purpose of waste audit?**
    Waste audit is required to understand the type and quantity of waste generated. It also helps in formulation of plan for segregation handling and management.

12. **What important functions the biomedical waste (BMW) audit serves?**
    The following functions (BMW) audit serves are—
    - It define the source of waste
    - The quantity generated from each source
    - The type of waste generated
    - It brings out the gaps in waste management process
    - It highlights the aspects of waste management process which require improvements or any alteration to make it more purposeful.

- The audit process helps in setting up targets so as to achieve waste reduction
- The waste audit improves the knowledge, and attitude of employees towards BMW management.

13. **What are the main managerial issues in BMWM?**
    - Waste recognition
    - Recognition of waste generation
    - Recognizing the cause of generation of particular type of waste
    - Planning of corrective action.

14. **What should be the contents of BMWM policy?**
    The policy must contain the following as mandatory contents. Policies and procedures should be made available and include the following:
    - Strategies for minimizing the quantities of biomedical waste generated and disposed off.
    - Methods of segregating, packaging, labeling, inhouse moving, storing, transporting and treating and final disposal if inhouse facility available otherwise steps up to transportation is enough because once it is transported to common biomedical waste treatment facility (CBMTF) then responsibility lies with the treatment facility owner.
    - Methods for keeping records of the quantities of biomedical waste generated, treated, and disposed.
    - List of all applicable regulations and legislation concerning biomedical waste as per state and central pollution control boards.
    - List of staff who is responsible for managing biomedical waste in the event of an accident or spill.
    - Provision for regular, ongoing staff training regarding handling and potential hazards of biomedical waste if not managed scientifically.

15. **What are the objectives of BMWM guidelines?**
    The objective of BMWM guidelines are:
    - To provide uniform standards for the segregation, transportation, storarge, treatment and final disposal of infectious or potentially infectious biomedical waste.
    - To mitigate the incidence of healthcare worker (HCW) and general population from contacting a disease or injury from biomedical waste.

- To provide guidance to the healthcare system on the opportunities for waste minimization and the reduction of environmental contamination from biomedical waste.

16. **What is the difference between dispensaries and clinics?**

    Dispensary—this is a facility which is designed to offer outpatient services with many doctors providing their services. This is also called polyclinic.

    Clinics—these are the facilities which are designed to offer outpatient services with only one doctor who is providing services to patients.

17. **What are the major biomedical waste management concerns for waste management officer?**

    All issues related to BMW should be of concern, however major concerns are:
    - What is quantum of waste per bed and what are the determinants for such quantum of waste?
    - What is the infectious potential of the waste generated?
    - What is the proportion of the infectious waste in total waste generated?
    - What are the current practices adopted by the healthcare facility in managing the biomedical waste?
    - What is proportion of polyvinyl chloride (PVC) containing items in the total waste?
    - What is the cost involvement for biohazards and environmental hazards and what are the alternatives available to reduce cost for the same?

18. **What are the benefits of methodical waste management?**
    - Scientific handling of waste
    - Efficient collection of waste
    - Economic disposal of waste
    - Elimination of occupational hazards related to waste.

19. **What are the characteristics of audit team?**
    - Team should be multidisciplinary
    - Every member should have authorized access to all staff member and departments of the hospital
    - Has expertize in waste management practices.

20. **During waste survey what should be the frequency of data collection?**
    - Wards, outpatient department (OPD), intensive care unit (ICU), casualty, laboratory—every shift.

- Operation theater (OT), dialysis, radiation unit—every procedure
- Laboratory chemical, liquid waste—before each discard into drain.
- Pharmacy, surrounding, administrative area, cleaning and washing water using flow meter, incinerator ash—once a day
- Kitchen—twice a day.

21. **What are the prerequisite of effective survey?**
    - The survey team should be dedicated towards their aim
    - No portion of total waste be missed out
    - Team should take each and every detail related to waste
    - A suitable place should be earmarked to carryout.

22. **What should be the minimum period for carrying out survey?**
    3-4 days a week every 4-6 weeks.

23. **What should be the frequency of waste survey in the healthcare facility?**
    It is of paramount importance that the staff who has been assigned duty of waste survey do not deviate from the set protocol of the organization.

Unit/department	Frequency of survey (data collection)
Operation theater	After each operation or surgical procedure
Intensive care units	Each shift
Emergency department	Each shift
Laboratory	Each shift
Dialysis unit	After each procedure
Ward (each ward need to be surveyed separately)	Each shift
Radiation unit	After each procedure
Outpatient department	Each shift
Pharmacy	Once a day
Central store	Once a day
Administrative units	Once a day
Kitchen	Twice a day
Surroundings of the healthcare facility	Once a day

24. **What are the specifications for the containers used for BMW collection?**
    Followings are the specifications for the container/bags which are used for BMW collection:
    - It should be sturdy enough to sustain the volume and weight of the waste without getting damaged.
    - The container should not have leak or puncture.
    - Sharps should be place in puncture proof containers and before putting sharps into container they should be mutilated.
    - Container should preferably have foot operated cover.
    - In case plastic bags are being used then these should be fitted in such a manner that they do not slipped when the cover of container is operated.
    - Container or bag should have three-fourth mark so that staff is aware not to fill more than that mark thus preventing spilling of the waste.

25. **What do you understand by waste tracking?**
    This is the process of documentation of the movement of the waste from the place of generation to the place of final disposal.

26. **What are the advantages of waste tracking?**
    - Proper monitoring of waste management program
    - Pinpointing the responsibility and liability
    - Records of quantities and type of waste generated, treated and disposed
    - Help in finding out the gaps in the process.

27. **How waste management process can be understood through the flowchart or process charts?**
    These charts are used to understand the management process from the step of waste generation to waste disposal.
    - Fishbone chart
    - Process flowchart.

28. **What the Fishbone chart depicts?**
    This is also known as Ishikawa or cause and effect diagram. It is called fishbone because it looks like that. This chart is used to improve the performance of the work flow and team by virtue of determining potential root cause of the problem.

29. **How process flowchart helps in management of biomedical waste?**

This chart or diagram gives idea about each and every step in the complete process of operations. This diagram makes it very easy to visualize the whole process. The process can be improved by adding, combining or changing the step in the flowchart.

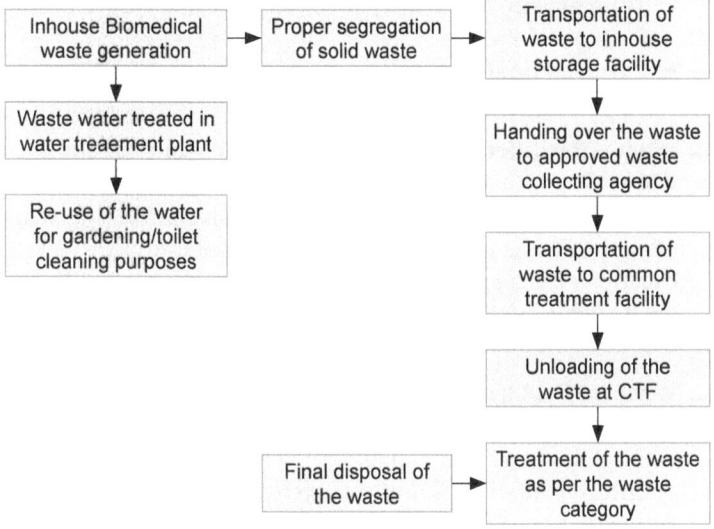

Flowchart: Biomedical waste management. (CTF: common treatment facility)

30. **Who do you mean by extended producer responsibility?**
    This is the part of waste minimization program in which producer of the product is responsible for the recovery of that particular product in case of not used/expired from date of manufacture, etc.

31. **What are other components of waste minimization?**
    - Product substitution (more ecofriendly product)
    - Product change to get more user-friendly product
    - Procedural change in patient care to minimize the waste generation
    - Preference for reusable items.

32. **What steps a healthcare facility should take to prepare a waste management plan?**
    - Have commitment to deliver the highest standard of patient care and safety of employee
    - Conduct baseline waste audit
    - Prepare waste minimization policy
    - Concentrate on 3'R' recycle, reduce and reuse concepts

- Take detailed accounts of segregation, storage, transport, treatment and disposal
- Comply with regulatory requirement of waste management
- Prepare risk management strategies
- Training and development of all who are involved in hospital facility and BMWM
- Ensure in time feedback on various components of plan
- Update regularly and periodically.

33. What is the difference between waste management and waste disposal?

Waste management: It is a comprehensive process in which all steps of waste management are well planned and strictly executed. It is a problem solver.

Waste disposal: Unplanned process in which waste is disposed off in discriminately. It is problem creator.

34. What is PDCA cycle?

It is a system to monitor systemic management of waste consisting of four steps—plan - do - check - act. It is also known as PDSA—Plan - Do - Study - Act cycle. PDCA cycle was originally conceived by Walter Shewhart in 1930 and later adapted by W Edward Deming in 1950, hence, also known as Deming cycle.

35. What are the details of each component?

Plan	Do	Check	Act
Establish policy based on requirement	Carry out changes initially on small scale by leading examples and showing commitments	Periodic review of objectives	If expected results are obtained then complexity of cycle is increased
Define objectives aimed at improvement	Collect data thoroughly	Results analyzed and trend of change is monitored	If no expected results then repeat the cycle till objective is achieved
Plan and provide resources	Implement corrective actions	This step is also called assessment step	Document the process and revise plan
Develop implementation of plan	Communicate action to be taken to all concerned		

36. **What are the objectives of PDCA cycle?**
    - To generate thought among healthcare workers that BMWM is continuous process
    - Effective achievement of BMWM.

37. **What is ramp of improvement?**
    It is upward going ramp of complexity on which once the PDCA's objective achieved then leading to new and slightly complex project in order to achieve continual improvement (Fig. 8.1).

38. **Mention the advantages of PDCA cycle?**
    - Immediacy, accuracy and ease of the application of the system
    - It gives competitive edge to organization

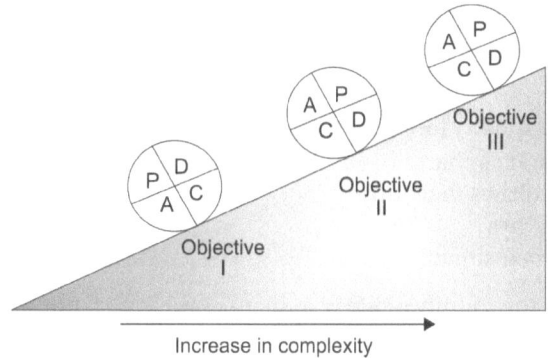

Fig. 8.1: Ramp of improvement.

   - It helps to determine the improvement priorities
   - It helps to apply measurement and charts to track process performance results.
   - It helps to create and deploy high performance process improvement team.

39. **What are the key elements for improvement in BMWM?**
    - Building up a comprehensive system for waste management
    - Resource allocation
    - Addressing responsibilities and authorities
    - Handling and disposal.

40. **What type of waste audit can be done?**
    There are two types of waste audit:
    1. Internal waste audit: Done by hospital senior staff
    2. External audit: Carried out by some designated external agencies.

41. **Can six sigma approach be applied in hospital waste management?**
    Yes

42. **How six sigma approach will be effective in BMW management?**
    Because:
    - It is a scientific, innovative and strategic way of doing work
    - The decisions are system based not the individual based
    - It reduces the defects in the systems.

43. **What are the advantages of six sigma approach?**
    - It is a teamwork
    - It is a continuous process
    - It will reduce the incidences of occupational injuries and diseases
    - Achievement of healthy environment.

44. **What quality tools can be used in hospital waste management?**
    - Parato's chart
    - Ishikawa diagram
    - 5 Whys
    - Process maps.

45. **How the quality of BMW management can be improved?**
    The elimination of the defects in the process of BMWM will improve the waste management process. The elimination of the defects can be achieved by:
    - Training of the staff dealing with the waste generation and waste disposal process
    - Brainstorming of the staff members
    - Mistake proofing.

46. **How ISO 14001 is related to hospital waste management?**
    ISO 14001 is related to environment management and hospital being responsible for the proper waste management. This includes:
    - Recognition of team leader for waste management
    - Improved risk management profile
    - Self-regulation
    - Decrease in release of airborne contaminants
    - Employee awareness toward environment.

47. What is EPP?

It means environmentally preferable purchasing and it consists of sourcing the products which are:
- Less toxic
- Reusable
- Leave less residue or waste behind when used
- Not having excessive packaging material.

48. What is PROFIT model of quality improvement?

P—problem identification
R—root cause identification and analysis
O—optimal solution based on root cause(s)
F—finalize how to implement corrective actions
I—implementation of corrective actions
T—tracking of effectiveness of implementation and verification of achievements of desired results.

PROFIT is the mnemonic for the group of actions which are taken for the quality improvement.

49. What are the strategic recommendations for improving hospital waste management?

- Define the problem clearly in waste management
- Focus on segregation
- Institute sharp management practices
- Keep focus on reduction of generation of waste
- Ensure worker's safety through protective equipment, education and training
- Secured collection and transportation
- Plan and policies for ensuring clarity and continuity of management practices
- Invest in employees training and ecofriendly waste treatment and disposal technologies
- Development of infrastructure for safe disposal and recycling of hazardous and general waste.

50. Is there any need of having BMW management committee in healthcare facility?

Yes, there is a need of BMW management committee in hospitals and composition of such committee should be:
Chairman—head of the institute

Vice chairman—microbiologist
Members—representatives from various departments like operations, housekeeping, stores, security, medical and nursing
Convener—infection control nurse.

51. **What are the role and responsibilities of BMW management committee?**

    BMW management committee is mainly responsible for:
    - Formulation of standard operating procedures (SOPs) regarding BMW management in the organization
    - Awareness generation among staff, patient and visitors regarding BMW and it's impact on health
    - Keep a vigil on supply of resources required for proper management of waste
    - Periodic meeting with the BMW management team and get feedback and take actions as deemed fit
    - Have meeting on assigned scheduled to review the waste management process in the organization.

52. **What is the advantage of Polyolefin intravenous (IV) bags over polyvinyl chloride (PVC) IV bags?**

    Polyolefin IV bags does not contain chlorine hence it has less potential to produce dioxin on incineration which PVC produces. Thus avoidance of environmental pollution by polyolefin is the advantage over PVC.

53. **What is the meaning of halogenated plastic and how it is different from nonhalogenated plastic?**

    Halogenated plastic is a type of plastic that contains halogen atoms, such as chlorine, bromine, fluorine, iodine, etc. Combustion of these types of plastic materials results in the generation of acid gases, such as hydrogen chloride. Examples of halogenated plastic—PVC and fluorocarbon compounds like Teflon.

    Nonhalogenated plastic is a type of plastics that does not contain atoms of halogen atoms in its constitution. Examples—polyethylene, polycarbonate and polystyrene.

54. **What is green procurement policy and what is the challenge in implementing it in healthcare facility?**

    Procurement of the products which will be used for patient care and as a waste they are environmentally preferable thus causing minimal environmental pollution. This is called green procurement policy.

Staff responsible for purchase and procurement comes from varied background hence having different frame of mind and thought process. In healthcare organization the environmental background and/or training is not being the prerequisite for their recruitment is responsible for environmentally unfriendly products. Under the umbrella of green purchase policy the waste minimization can be achieved by procuring reusable products which can be easily disinfected and reused or purchase of chlorine and/or mercury free products.

55. **How saving in cost of waste management can be achieved?**

   The saving in cost of waste management can be achieved by reduction in the cost associated with clinical waste and this reduction can be achieved by:
   - Reducing the volume of clinical waste produced
   - Reducing the unit cost of disposal items used in patient care, the unit cost of disposal item depends on the contract price which has been negotiated by purchase department with vendors.

56. **What is Sanpro medical waste?**

   The term Sanpro is a description not classification and it includes the items used for disposal of feces, urine and other bodily secretions and excretions but which does not contain identifiable blood and human tissue. Sanpro waste generated in hospital will treated as clinical waste but when generated at home it is treated as domestic waste.

57. **What is the annual quantum of hospital waste in India?**

   The quantum of hospital waste in India is around 3 million every year and amount is expected to grow at 8% annually.

58. **What is personal protective equipment (PPE) program?**

   This is the written guidelines which every healthcare should have in its possession. This includes:
   - Organization's policy statement
   - Particular healthcare organization's, local, state level and national level relevant regulations
   - Policies, procedures and SOPs
   - Hazard identification

- Selection and use of PPE
- Maintenance and decontamination of PPE
- Training.

59. **What are the objectives of PPE program?**

    The PPE program serves two objectives:
    1. To protect wearer from any health hazard and provide safety
    2. To prevent injury to wearer from incorrect use and/or malfunction of PPE's use.

60. **What is site safety plan?**

    It is the plan which establishes policies and procedures in order to protect the hospital and healthcare facility biomedical waste handlers and community population from potential hazards posed by the waste sites inside and outside hospital, respectively. The plan also provides measures so as to minimize injuries and accidents that may occur while working at waste sites.

61. **What are the challenges to biomedical waste management practices in India?**

    India being vastly diverse country in various widely differing political, economical and demographic aspects, therefore putting forward challenges to the proper biomedical waste management practices. Inadvertent disposal of such environmentally unfriendly waste lead to tremendous public health problem leading to filing of several public interest litigations (PILs) exerting pressure on government to enact a law which will govern healthcare waste management. The major challenges identified but not limited to are:

    - **Lack of segregation practices:** Segregation practice at the site of waste generation prevents mixing of noninfectious waste with infectious waste. Lack of segregation practices significantly increases the quantity of infectious medical waste as mixing makes the entire mass potentially infectious. In Indian hospital and healthcare institutions this is observed at all level from waste generator to handlers thus losing the importance of segregation.
    - **Lack of proper operational strategy:** Operational plans for BMWM should include the capacity and location of storage containers, frequency of collection for various types of wastes and schedule of activities. Infectious wastes need to be stored

in the designated color-coded, leak-proof containers and can be disinfected/sterilized by the available effective facility in the hospital. Transportation of waste within the hospital is to be carried out in closed handcarts to avoid spillage of waste. After local disinfection/sterilization the waste is transported to a common treatment facility. However the fact is that wastes are generally collected in mixed forms, transported in open carts resulting in spillage and waste sharps are discarded without disinfection and mutilation resulting in being reused leading to spread of infection.

- **Poor regulative measures:** In India, Central Pollution Control Board and the State Pollution Control Boards, the agencies responsible to enforce these rules in hospitals are at one hand lacking adequate power and on the other hand there is no commitment. As a result, most of the large hospitals have not complied with these rules even after expiry of new deadlines. Even the regulatory authorities have to take the blame for not doing enough to ensure implementation. There is lack of coordination between the regulatory authorities and other departments. Rules have not been publicized as widely as required resulting in smaller cities housing. Small high care unit (HCUs) may not be fully aware of these rules.
- **Lack of green procurement policy:** Personnel responsible for procuring healthcare products and services (materials managers or purchasing agents) in hospitals come from different backgrounds. Environmental background or training is not a prerequisite for the selection and appointment of these staff members. Waste minimization can be achieved by purchasing reusable items made of glass and metals which can be disinfected and reused. For example, a polyolefin IV bag does not contain chlorine, so it has less potential to produce dioxins through incineration than an IV bag containing PVC. Another example is the replacement of mercury thermometers with mercury free thermometers. Healthcare units should stimulate the purchase of environmentally preferable products by changing purchase policies.
- **Waste picking and reusing:** Reuse of plastic syringes and other plastic material has been a thriving business of billions of Indian Rupees. It is estimated that more than one million people are engaged in rag picking. Lucrative monetary returns

and lack of awareness about the problems associated with biomedical wastes encourage waste picking and reusing activities. The waste from waste handlers goes to rag pickers who sale these waste to the packaging outlets situated in slum, from there packed material goes to the medical shop, and finally sold to the unsuspecting patients or their relatives at cheaper prices.

- **Lack of top management commitment:** Governments and private healthcare providers have gone in for one type of option for treatment of the waste and that is incineration. No healthcare provider has undertaken a baseline survey to collect data regarding quantum of waste and its type being generated, nor about the waste generation points in its premises. Secondly budgetary support being poor for this activity leading to ignorance towards these rules for the monetary consideration. Top management in most of Indian hospitals is showing inertia in dealing with the waste problem.

- **Lack of adequate facilities:** Guanine efforts to provide facilities for storage, collection, treatment and disposal of healthcare wastes as well as appropriate technologies have so far been limited in India and to add to this there is deficiency of availability of sanitary landfills as well. Therefore, the biomedical waste are openly dumped into the open bins on the road sides, low lying area or they are directed into the water bodies. There is also deficiency in innovations in disposal options in accordance to the complexity of healthcare waste.

- **Lack of institutional arrangements:** Management of healthcare waste depends on the input from the administration and active participation by trained staff in segregation, storage, collection, transportation, treatment and disposal. In India personnel responsible for these activities are mainly ward attendants and other supporting staff. A committee consisting of the head of the establishment, all the departmental heads, hospital superintendents, nursing superintendents and hospital engineers should be formed with a waste management officer who would be advised by an environmental control advisor and an infection control advisor is required for proper waste management purposes. Studies showed lack of such kind in hospital waste management committee or

documented waste management plan and disposal policy in Indian hospitals.
- **Financial constraints:** To have independent waste treatment systems in HCUs, financial provision is necessary for capital and recurring expenditure. As generally seen a separate allocation of funds for waste management is not found in Indian hospitals. This resulting in smaller HCUs ignore waste management practices. In Indian subcontinent it is estimated that expenditure of INR 3,000–4,000 per tonne of hospital waste is required. Additionally funds are required for conducting training and awareness programs for staffs.
- **Inadequate awareness and training programs:** Awareness of appropriate handling and disposal of healthcare wastes among health personnel is a priority; it is essential that everyone should know the potential health hazards. Regular programs will help to prevent exposure of healthcare wastes and related hazards. Poster exhibition, proper labeling, and explanation by staff are effective methods. Seminars and workshops, and participation in training courses are also essential. Management in most of Indian hospitals is not aware of cost savings achieved due to good waste management practices. It has also been estimated that disposal savings between 40% and 70% could be realised through the implementation of a healthcare waste reduction program.
- **Reluctance to change and adoption:** Though now alternative technologies are permitted as per the biomedical Rules, it takes a long time to change the mindset of the people. Even now most of the healthcare providers and decision-making authorities talk of incinerator only although autoclaves and other advanced waste handling equipments are available. Indiscriminate throwing of the waste is still seen in most of the hospitals and the waste handlers still are without protective clothing and gears. There is hardly any change in the applied knowledge and awareness seen in Indian hospitals.
- **Inadequate pressure from societies:** Previous studies show that pressure from various Environmental advocacy groups forces, organizations to seriously think about their environmental management programs which is lacking in the case of Indian organizations. There is no doubt in the mind of any educated or enlightened person that improper hospital

waste management is the source of many communicable and infectious diseases. But when it comes to doing anything there is a complete lack of will, and there is a lackadaisical attitude towards the problem.

62. **What is green supply chain management (GSCM)?**

Green supply chain management can be defined as integrating environmental thinking into supply-chain management. The concept includes product design, material sourcing and selection, along with post use management of the product.

GSCM actually integrates social concerns indicating that economic systems are contained in social systems which are in turn contained in ecological systems.

It is a sustainable way to achieve dual purpose, increase in efficiency as well as lowering in cost by reducing the disposal amount of waste material with the help of recycle, repair and remanufacture operations. This way the concept is sustainable for the environment because materials will not be left on the ground while giving harm to the environment.

It can be summarized as a part of the environmental awareness approach, process, enabling to minimize negative environmental effects of supply chain management in the hospital and determine the activities so as to use optimum source and to reduce complexity.

63. **What are the benefits of GSCM?**

In green hospitals by using green supply chain management following benefits can be achieved. These are divided in to three categories which are as follows:

Environments benefits	Social benefits	Economical benefits
Reduction in waste	Reduced community effect	Reduced operational cost
Reduction in air emissions	Health promotion	Increased revenue, i.e. improved bottom line revenue
Increased energy efficiency	Improved patient satisfaction	Increased material utilization
Reduction in pollution level		Enhanced customer service

Chapter 9

New Concept in Biomedical Waste Management

1. **What is 3R?**
   - Reduce
   - Recycle
   - Reuse.

2. **What is difference between recycle and reuse?**
   Recycle: Process of using waste products as a raw material to produce either similar material or other material. Examples of recycle product to new product:
   - Glass → Glass
   - Paper → Paper, cardboard
   - Plastic → Plastic

   Reuse: Process of using the waste product for the same purpose for which it was originally used.
   Glass syringe → used → washed and sterilized → Reuse.

3. **What are the benefits of waste minimization?**
   - Economic reduction of waste generated
   - Efficient handling of waste
   - Economic disposal
   - Reduction in health hazards.

4. **What is waste to energy concept?**
   This is the concept of regeneration of energy from the waste either in the form of fuel or gas.

5. **What is the concept of sustainable hospital?**
   The concept of sustainable hospital concepts are as follows:
   - Efficient biomedical waste management
   - Elimination of environmental or occupational hazards

- Maintenance of total quality in patient care
- Cost contaminant.

6. **Define Green purchasing.**
   This is the system of purchasing hospital items which are:
   - Nontoxic
   - Environmental friendly
   - More energy efficient
   - Highly recyclable
   - Safer for patient and staff.

7. **What is zero waste?**
   It is the logical planning approach incorporating principles of effective human and material resource utilization to convert discards into efficient form of energy.

   Waste of one type acts as resource for the other type new product.
   Waste paper: Cardboard boxes.
   Nature makes no waste: It is the invention of human beings.

8. **What are the strategies to achieve zero waste?**
   - Adopt resource management plan because it is easier to manage the resource than waste
   - Make 3R the heart of the plan
   - Composting of the waste
   - Make participative and meaningful program for waste management
   - Zero waste certification as an incentive
   - Development of market for recyclable items
   - Top level management involvement
   - Extended responsibility of manufacturer
   - Development of toxic release inventory to educate those who are concerned with waste management
   - Focusing on renewable resources so as to get and do more with less resources.

9. **What are end results of zero waste?**
   - Reduced occupational risks to employees
   - Reduce risk to environment
   - Elimination of toxins from environment
   - Cost contaminant.

10. **Can solar energy be utilized in BMWM.**
    Yes:
    - Box type solar cooker
    - Portable autoclave powered by solar energy.

11. **How waste minimization be achieved in day-to-day practice?**
    - Use material in least required quantity and only when it is absolutely essential
    - Prepare group purchasing or bulk purchasing
    - Purchase ecofriendly/biodegradable material
    - More preference to reusable item
    - Bulk/expiry/excess item to be returned to supplier/manufacturer as dealt in the initial contract.

12. **What is PATH?**
    It is a program which is called Programme for Appropriate Technology in Health (PATH). This is a partnership project between PATH and Andhra Pradesh government started. Having aim of creating a "Model Immunization Program" thus incorporating modern immunization system with new methods, policies and procedures. The pilot program was for 6 months. In the program the use of automatic disabled (AD) started in immunization program. Around one million syringes were used during the project period. The sharp and plastic components were collected, treated and disposed separately. Extensive training were given to all concerned staff. This project concluded that nonburn techniques can also be equally effective provided with proper training and motivation given to staff.

Chapter 10

Laws Related to Biomedical Waste Management

1. **What are biomedical waste (management and handling) rules, 1998?**

   These rules prescribed by Ministry of Environment and Forest as per the provisions contained in Sections 6, 8, and 25 of Environment (Protection) Act, 1986 in order to protect the environment from the pollutants produced by biomedical waste in any form. These rules have been amended two times first in 2000 and later in 2003.

   These rules were notified on 20th July 1998, however, draft rules were Gazetted on 16th Oct 1997 and public opinion and suggestions were invited within 60 days and they were considered before finalization of the rules. These rules provide uniform guidelines and code of practice for the whole nation.

   It is clearly mentioned in this rule that the 'occupier' (a person who has control over the concerned institution/premises) of an institution generating biomedical waste (e.g. hospital, nursing home, clinic, dispensary, veterinary institution, animal house, pathological laboratory, AYUSH, blood bank, etc.) shall be responsible for taking necessary steps to ensure that such waste is handled without any adverse effect to human health and the environment.

2. **What are hazardous substances?**

   There are substances or preparations which due to their physiochemical or chemical properties or handling liable to cause harm to human beings or other living creatures, plants, property or environment.

3. **What is authorization?**

   Permission granted by the prescribed authority for generation, collection, reception, storage, transportation, treatment, disposal and/or any other form of handling of biomedical waste in accordance with these rules and any guidelines issued by central government.

4. **Who are the occupiers?**

   Any institution generating biomedical waste includes hospital, clinic, dental clinic, laboratory, veterinary institution, animal house, nursing home, blood bank and others by any name who has control over the institution and/or its premises.

5. **What types of waste is taken by municipal body?**
   - General waste
   - Treated biomedical waste for disposal.

6. **Who laid down the standards for treatment technology of biomedical waste (BMW)?**

   Central pollution control board (CPCB).

7. **What is the period of authorization?**

   Initial authorization is given for 3 years including one year provisional authorization. Subsequent authorization is also granted for 3 years.

8. **Who are the prescribed authorities for States and Union territories?**

   For states—State Pollution Control Boards
   For Union Territories—Pollution Control Committees.

9. **What is prescribed authorities?**

   It is an authority which is prescribed by state/central government in order to get biomedical waste management (BMWM) rules implemented. For the states the state pollution control board is the prescribed authority while for union territories the pollution control committee are the prescribed authority.

10. **What is the period for application disposal for authorization?**

    Within 90 days from the date of receipt of application for authorization.

11. **What are the powers and responsibilities of prescribed authority?**

    The powers and responsibilities of the prescribed authority are:
    - Grant of authorization to the institutions covered under this rule
    - Implementing various provisions of this rule for proper management and handling of biomedical waste
    - Call for information in prescribed form as per Form 1
    - To make such enquiries as it deems fit
    - To conduct surveys, inspections and investigations for the purpose of implementation of this rule
    - To refuse grant of authorization. This has to be in writing and reasonable opportunity should be given to the applicant
    - To dispose of application of authorization within ninety days of receipt of application
    - To give a reasonable opportunity to the applicant before cancellation or suspension.

12. **What are powers/responsibilities of occupier?**

    The occupier/operator/applicant has the following powers/responsibilities:
    - Specific procedure of grant of authorization or its cancellation or suspension
    - To submit application in prescribed application form for authorization
    - To give all the relevant information's including necessary fee, as prescribed by the prescribed authority, for grant of authorization
    - To renew the authorization within the specified period
    - Refusal or suspension of authorization only when recorded in writing giving reasons
    - Automatic grant of authorization if the application not disposed by the prescribed authority within 90 days of receipt of the application, provided the application is complete in all respects
    - Authorization granted for three years including an initial trial period of 1 year from the date of issue
    - Provisional authorization may be granted by the prescribed authority for the trial period
    - Specific time limit for compliance of provisions of the BMW Rules 98.

13. **List out the duties of healthcare facility.**
    - Provide personal protective equipment (PPE) to healthcare workers
    - Report major accidents
    - Make available the annual report on its website
    - Inform the prescribed authority immediately if waste is not picked or retained for more than 48 hours
    - Establish a committee to review and meet once in every six months and the record of the minutes of the meetings of this committee and incorporate in annual report
    - Maintain all records for a period of 5 years
    - Conduct health check up at the time of induction and at least once in a year for all its health care workers
    - Maintain daily register and upload monthly records on website.

14. **Which occupiers are exempted from taking authorization?**
    Dispensaries, clinics, pathological labs and blood banks which are providing services to less than 1000 patients per month. However, they have to comply with rules for management of waste generated.

    No hospital or nursing home is exempted irrespective of bed strength and number of patients per month.

15. **When the annual report be submitted by the occupier?**
    Annual report should be submitted by the occupier to prescribed authority by 31st January every year who in turn sends it to CPCB by 31st March every year.

16. **What is the deadline for annual report as per Rules 2018?**
    All the health care facilities (any number of beds) shall make available the annual report on its website within a period of two years from the date of publication of Bio-Medical Waste Management (Amendment) Rules, 2018.

17. **What forms are used by occupiers?**
Form I	For application for authorization
Form II	For annual report
Form III	For accident report
Form IV	For authorization for operating a facility for collection
Form V	For application for filing appeal against order passed by prescribed authority.

18. **How many Schedules are there in BMW (management and handling) rules, 1998?**

Schedule I	Classification of biomedical waste in different categories
Schedule II	Types and color coding of the containers to be used for each category of BMW
Schedule III	Proforma for the label to be used on container/bags
Schedule IV	Proforma for the label for transport of waste container/bags
Schedule V	Standards for treatment and disposal of waste
Schedule VI	Deadlines for creation of waste treatment facilities.

19. **What are the 4 schedules and 5 forms new BMWM rules, 2016?**

Schedule I	BMW color coding, collection, treatment and disposal
Schedule II	Standards for treatment and disposal
Schedule III	Prescribed authorities and responsibilities
Schedule IV	Labels for BMW containers and bags
Form I	Accident reporting
Forms II and III	Application and authorization document
Form IV	Annual report
Form IV	Annual report by SPCB or AFMS to CPBB
Form V	Appeal

20. **What are the requirements for BMWM as per new guidelines of 2016?**

New requirements	Timeline for implementation	Remarks
Pretreatment of laboratory waste, microbiology waste, blood samples before giving to disposal	*Immediate effect	Within 2 years from date of issue for Principle BMW 2016 now extended to 27th March 2019
Phase out chlorinated bags, gloves, blood bags		
Training health care workers about handling of biomedical waste	*Immediate effect	Details of training to be submitted along with annual report

Contd...

Contd...

New requirements	Timeline for implementation	Remarks
Immunization of health care workers for hepatitis B and tetanus	With immediate effect	Records of vaccination to be maintained
Bar code system for bags or containers containing biomedical waste		Within 1 year from date of issue of Principle rules BMW 2016 now extended to 27th March 2019
Health checkup of health care workers during induction and annually thereafter	With immediate effect	Records to be maintained
Maintain and update biomedical waste management register and monthly report on website	With in 2 years from date of issue of Principle rule BMW-2016 rules, i.e. within 28th March 2018	On Compliance Portal in ESS
Major accidents to be reported along with annual report	Should be documented and reported	Nil
Maintain records of auto claving, microwaving, etc. for a period of five years	With immediate effect	Nil
Annual report on website		Within 2 years from date of issue of Principle Rules 2016 now extended to 16th March 2020
Setup BMW management committee, and meetings be done bi-annually. Minutes submitted in annual report	With immediate effect	

21. **What is the time deadline for establishing waste management facilities by occupiers as per the schedule VI?**

The deadline for time limit as per schedule VI of BMWM Rules was by 31 December 2002, for all hospitals and nursing homes.

22. **When appeal against the orders passed by the prescribed authority be done?**
    Within 30 days from the date on which the order communicated to the occupier. Beyond this time appeal can be entertained in case authority feels that appellant was prevented by sufficient cause from filling the appeal in time.

23. **What are minimum terms and conditions for authorization?**
    - Authorization shall comply with the provision given in rules.
    - Authorization letter or renewed authorization letter shall be produced for inspection on and when asked by person authorized by prescribed authority.
    - No change in personnel equipment or working conditions mentioned in application be done without prior permission from prescribed authority.
    - There should be no procedural change in BMWM without prior permission from prescribed authority.
    - Before closing down the facility prior permission of prescribed authority is essential.

24. **What is the minimum space requirement for waste management?**

S. No.	Hospital type	Free area required (in hectare)
1.	Nonbedded hospitals, clinical labs, bedded hospitals	0.02
2.	Less than 50 beds	0.25
3.	50–200	1.00
4.	More than 200	2.5
5.	Research center and diagnostic center	0.1

25. **How the charges are fixed for BMWM?**
    Charges in hospital are fixed as per bed per day basis and on approximate weight basis for other establishment where there are no beds.

26. **What are the prescribed regulatory authorities responsible for BMWM?**
    - Ministry of health and family welfare
    - Ministry of environment and forests
    - Director general of armed forces medical services

- Director General Health Services of respective states for central pollution control boards
- State pollution control boards
- Municipal authorities.

27. **Under which Act the non-compliance to Rules is punishable?**
    Non-compliance to Rules is punishable under Sections 16 and 17 of Environment (Protection) Act 1986. Punishment can be any or all of the following:
    - Imprisonment for 5 years extendable to 7 years
    - Fine upto ₹ 1 lakhs
    - Both of the above.

28. **What are the responsibilities of CPCB for BMWM?**
    - Monitoring of implementation
    - Preparation of codes, manuals and guidelines
    - Compilation of data
    - Monitoring of implementation of rules
    - Providing technical assistance to state pollution control boards.
    - Organizing CME
    - Laying down standards for:
        - Incinerator
        - Hydroclave
        - Autoclave
        - Microwave
    - Preparation of guidelines for:
        - Design and construction for incinerator
        - Common BMW treatment facility
        - Management of waste from universal immunization program.

29. **What are the responsibilities of state pollution control boards?**
    - Giving authorization for BMWM by facility
    - Renewal of authorization
    - Collection of annual reports
    - Periodic checking of facilities for compliance to Rules
    - Checking of all records maintained by occupier
    - Issuing notice for violating the norms of BMW disposal
    - Checking of various emission standards for incinerator and standards for liquid waste
    - Creating awareness among their own staff and other health care workers.

30. **What authorities have been empowered to government under Environment (Protection) Act, 1986?**

The authority is given to government to implement there rules under various sections of this Act:

Section 3 To undertake various steps for protection and improvement of the environment

Section 6 Government is empowered to make rules to regulate environmental pollution

Section 8 Waste handlers have to comply with procedural safeguards given in rules

Section 10 Authority to enter and inspect the premises handling and managing the waste

Section 15 Government can take punitive actions against the defaulters

Section 17 In case offender is any government department then head of the department is deemed to be guilty and liable for punishment accordingly.

31. **When biomedical waste (management and handling) rules 1998 were amended**

These Rules were first amended in year 2000 then 2003 now the draft proposal has been made ready 2011 and is with competent authorities for required changes as deemed fit.

32. **What are key provisions in biomedical waste management rules 2011?**

The new rules are more elaborate, stringent and several new provisions have been added to it. The rules are not applicable for radioactive waste, hazardous waste, municipal waste and battery waste which will be dealt under respective rules. The difference between Rules 1998 and 2011 are follows:

BMW (Management and Handling) Rules, 1998	BMW (Management and Handling) Rules, 2011
Occupiers with more than 1000 beds required to obtain authorization	Irrespective of bed strength or quantum of waste the occupier need to take authorization
Mention of duties of operated were not given	Duties of operator are listed
Waste was categories in 10 classes	Waste categorization is reduced to 8

Contd...

Contd...

BMW (Management and Handling) Rules, 1998	BMW (Management and Handling) Rules, 2011
Regarding treatment and disposal the rules were restricted to healthcare having facility of more than 1000 beds	All healthcare facilities irrespective of bed strength need to stick to treatment and disposal of waste
Format for annual report not available	Format for annual report appended with rules
Form VI (report of operator on healthcare facilities not handing over biomedical waste) absent	Form VI has been added to the rules

33. **When the amendments were done in BMW management Rules and what was the main objective of these amendments?**

    The biomedical waste (management and handling) Rules were amended twice in year 2000. First amendment was published on 6th March 2000 vide S.O. 210 (E) which second amendment was published on 2nd June 2000 vide Gazette Notification S.O. 545 (E). Third amendment was published on 17th September 2003 vide Gazette Notification S.O. 1069 (E).

    The main objective of these amendments are to ensure proper and in a scientific way segregation, collection, transportation and disposal of the infectious BMW so as to provide safeguard to community health.

34. **What is the main thrust of amended BMW rules 2018?**

    The amended rules stipulate that generators of biomedical waste (hospitals, nursing homes, clinics, and dispensaries) will not use chlorinated plastic bags and gloves beyond March 27, 2019 in medical applications to save the environment. Only exemption is blood bags which are not to be phase out as per the amended BMW rules, 2018.

35. **Is municipal body responsible for collection and treatment of biomedical waste?**

    The municipal body is not responsible to collect and transport untreated biomedical wastes generated in any healthcare facility of their area while it is the responsibility of occupier of the healthcare units. Municipal body will collect and dispose the duly treated BMW for disposal at municipal dump site.

36. **How the notice of offense is given to occupier?**
    - Notice is given in Form IV and copy to different authority in state/UT.
        If offence has taken place in state:
        – State pollution control board
        – Environment secretary in State Govt
        – Secretary in Ministry of E and F
        If offence has taken place in UT:
        – Central pollution control board
        – Secretary in Ministry of E and F
    - Notice is sent by registered post with acknowledgement due (Registered AD).
    - A period of 60 days as mentioned in Clause (b) of Section 19 of Environment (Protection) Act 1986, be calculated from the date it is first received by one of the authorities mentioned above.

37. **What is the coverage area for CBWTF ?**
    - It extends its facility upto 10,000 beds within area of radius of 150 km.
    - Beyond 150 km, another unit is to be established.

38. **What treatment facilities should be made available at CBWTF?**
    - Autoclave/Hydroclave because more stress is given on non-burn techniques
    - Microwave
    - Incinerator with APCD
    - Shredder
    - Sharp pit
    - Secured landfill
    - Effluent treatment plant
    - Washing facilities
    - Water pumps, storage, air compressors
    - Generator for electricity.

39. **What is the machinery required for establishing the CWTF?**

Requirement	Quantity
Incinerator	Two
Autoclave	One
Shredder	One (optional Two)

Contd...

Requirement	Quantity
Microwave	One (optional)
Effluent treatment plant	One
Chimney for incinerator exhaust	One (height minimum 30 meters)
Water pump	One
Air compressor	One
Electricity Generator	One
Storage room	One
Waste transportation vehicle cleaning equipment	One

40. **What are the operating standards for incinerators?**

$$CE = \frac{\% CO_2}{\% CO_2 \times \% CO} \times 100$$

- Combustion efficiency shall be at least 99%
- Temp of binary chamber 800 + 50°C
- Temp of secondary chamber 1050 + 50°C with gas residence time at least one second and minimum 3% oxygen in stock gas
- Only low sulphur diesel shall be used
- Minimum stake height for incinerator should be 30 meters
- Chlorinated plastic, toxic metals should not incinerated
- Waste should not be chemically pretreated with chlorinated disinfectant.

41. **What are the emission standards for incinerators?**

Incinerators parameters	Concentration mg/Nm³ at 12% CO_2 correction
Particulate matter	150
Nitrogen oxides	450
Hydrogen chloride	50
Volatile organic compounds in incinerator ash	Less than 0.1%
Particulate matter	150
Nitrogen oxides	450
Hydrogen chloride	50
Volatile organic compounds in incinerator ash	Less than 0.1%

42. **What are the standards for incinerators at CBWTF?**
    - Capacity minimum 50 kg/hr
    - Separate burners for primary and secondary chambers with automatic on/off switch to avoid fluctuation in temperature
    - Flame in primary chamber point towards waste while in secondary chamber the gases passes through flames (Fig. 10.1).

    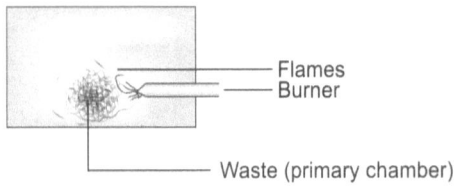

    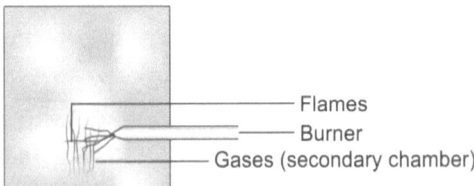

    Fig. 10.1: Flames in chamber.

    - Chambers should be lined with refractory and insulation bricks with 11-12 cm thickness.
    - Incinerator should have emergency went and should be opened only in case of emergency.
    - Around incinerator there should be a clear area of 1.5 m all around between incinerator and room wall.
    - Stock emission monitoring and incinerator ash analysis should be done quarterly and record should be maintained by operator.

43. **What is the new policy on incinerator establishment?**
    - Incinerator should be allowed only at CBMWT facility only
    - Installation of individual incinerator in healthcare facility shall be discouraged as far as possible however approval can be granted only in certain inevitable situations where no other option is feasible.

44. **What are the design criteria for better performance of incinerator?**

The incinerator is one of the main stay in BMW management and major part of the waste is treated through this mean. For the optimum functioning of the incinerator, it needs to be designed in such a manner that it works efficiently and for the same criteria have been laid down:
- The incinerator should be designed in such a manner that it take the capacity of more than 50 Kg per hour of incineration and for this minimum hearth are should be 8 sq ft along with this the minimum flow of flue gas in secondary chamber shall be 0.6 m^3/second at 1050°C.
- Each incinerator must have air pollution control system along with it.
- Preferably there should be double chamber incinerator as this is more efficient and air pollution is minimal on account of minimal particulate matter emission. Facility should follow the "controlled air incineration principle".
- The size of opening of the primary chamber should be large enough than the size of the waste bag which will be fed in to the chamber.
- The volume of the primary chamber should be at least five times of the expected volume of the batch.
- The inside of top and side corners of primary and secondary chambers should prefereably be rounded so as to avoid formation of dead zones/black pockets.
- Presence of negative water column shall be maintained and provision should be there to measure water column pressure.
- The chamber should strictly be fed as per manufacture's instruction.
- The secondary chamber should be designed in such a manner that residence time for gas flow remains for one second.
- The lining of chamber should be such that it sustain the minimum temperature of 1000°C and 1200°C in primary and secondary chamber respectively. The refractory bricks should have minimum of 155 mm thickness.
- The thickness of outer steel place should be about 5 mm and made of mild steel. The outer surface of steel plate is painted with heat resistant aluminum paint which can withstand a temperature of 250°C with proper surface preparation.

- Refractory lining of hot duct shall be done with refractory castable and insulating castable of minimum 45 mm and 80 mm thickness.
- Ceramic wool should be used at hot duct flanges and expansion joints.
- Waste should be fed through automatic feeding device. The system should be able to prevent operator from direct exposure of incinerator environment, prevent leakage of gases and avoid heaping of waste at one place and spread the waste in chamber equally.
- There should be separate burner for primary as well as secondary chamber. The burner should be able to raise the temperature of primary and secondary chamber to $850 \pm 50°C$ and $1050 \pm 50°C$. The desired temperature should reach within 60 minutes prior to charging the waste.
- Chamber burner should have automatic on/off system in accordance with desired temperature of incinerator chamber.
- Burner should have spark igniter and main burner.
- Appropriate flame safeguard and flame view observation support need to be installed.
- Specification about flame burner is that
    - Flame should be directed towards the center of the hearth
    - Flame should be long enough so that it touches waste however does not intrude the walls of incinerator.
    - The position of secondary chamber burner should be such that flue gas passes through the flames.
- Incinerator should have programmable logic control system (PLC) so as to prevent:
    - Charging of the chambers with waste until desired temperature is attained in both chambers.
    - Waste charging in case there are unsafe circumstances related to incinerator like very high or low temperature, nonworking of fan and recirculation pump, very high temperature of flue gases at outlet of air pollution control unit.
- Incinerator should have emergency vent.
- The chimney should have approximately 3 mm thick lining of heavy duty rubber so as to prevent corrosion from acids and oxygen in flue gases.

- There should be clear area of minimum 1.5 meters all around incinerator to wall of the room.

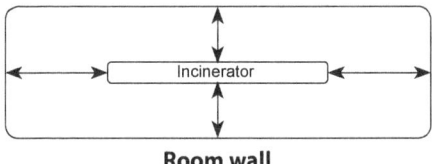

Room wall

- Waste store room must be adjacent to incinerator and should be well ventilated.
- The floor and inner walls of storage room and incinerator shall have outer covering of impervious and glazed material thus avoiding moisture retention and facilitating cleaning.
- The ash produced in incinerator shall be stored in sturdy container which can be tightly closed. Eventually this ash should be disposed off securely.
- Incinerator should be operated by a skilled and experience staff along with one assistant.
- All the records related to waste and incinerator specification should be maintained and updated regularly.
- Incinerator operator should be provided with all protective gears and should periodically undergo thorough medical checkups.
- All adverse events should be immediately intimated to competent authorities and records of such event maintained. Events should be analysed and appropriate CAPA (Corrective Action and Preventive Action) must be placed at the earliest.

45. **What are the specifications about high pressure venturi scrubber system?**
    - The system should be made up of stainless steel. It can also be made of mild steel and having lining of acid resistant bricks to prevent acid corrosion.
    - The system shall have minimum pressure drop of 350 mm WC (water column) so as to achieve prescribe emission limits. At the outlet of venturi system the temperature of flue gases should be dropped to 70–80° C so as to ensure saturation of flue gases.
    - The pH of scrubbing liquid must be above 6.5 and this is achieved by adding caustic soda solution to it.

- The system should be followed by centrifugal type droplet separator which removes water droplets from flue gases.
- The circulation speed of scrubbing medium should be kept at approximately 2.25 liters/cubic meters of flue gases at venture outlet.
- Waste water and stack emission should be handled as per the requirement of BMW management and handling rules.

46. **What are the standards for liquid waste generated from facility?**

pH	6.5 – 9.0
Suspendable solids	100 mg/L
Oil and grease	10 mg/L
Biological oxygen demand	30 mg/L
Chemical oxygen demand	250 mg/L
Bioassay test	90% survival of fish after 96 hr in 100% affluent

These parameters are applicable to hospitals which are:
- Connected to sewers without terminal sewage treatment plant
- Not connected to public sewers.

47. **What is the timeline for installing STP for hospital/healthcare facilities having bed strength less than 10?**

Hospitals/Health Care Facilities having less than ten beds shall have to install Sewage Treatment Plant by the 31st December, 2019. Non-bedded occupiers shall dispose infectious liquid wastes only after treatment by disinfection as per Schedule – II (6) of the principal rules.

48. **What are the operating standards for waste treatment autoclave?**

Vacuum type

Temperature	Pressure	Residence time
121°C	15 psi	45 min
135°C	31 psi	30 min

Gravity type

Temperature	Pressure	Residence time
121°C	15 psi	60 min
135°C	31 psi	45 min
149°C	52 psi	30 min

49. **How the autoclaving of waste is validated?**
    - By chemical strip indicator which changes its color when certain temperature is achieved. For adequate autoclave it is essential to use more than one strip at different locations.
    - By spore testing using *Bacillus stearothermophilus* spores in the form of vial or strips (1×10 spores/ml). Appropriate autoclaving will kill the spores.

50. **What spores testing is used in case of microwave?**
    Spores of *Bacillus subtilis* (either vials or strips having 1×10^4 spores/ml).

51. **What precautions to be taken while dealing with radioactive waste?**
    - Radioactive waste should not be disposed in regular trash or poured in drains
    - Use short lived isotopes whenever possible
    - Use specially designed area for storage of radioactive waste
    - Monitor closely
    - Take help of experts as and when needed.

52. **How the sampling of the liquid waste is done?**
    It is done by designated person who is empowered to take sample. The sample is divided into 3 equal parts.
    One portion handed over to facility with acknowledgement.
    Second portion sent forthwith to environment laboratory for analysis.
    Third portion is retained by officer to be produced in court in case any proceeding is instructed in court of law.
    The samples are marked and sealed by the person who has taken the samples and also by the facility from where the sample has been taken.

53. **Where deep burial is the method of choice for Category 1 and 2?**
    It is the method of choice for Category 1 and 2 wastes only in cities having less than 5 lakh populations.

54. **What should be minimum specification for shredder?**
    - Should need minimum maintenance
    - Should have electrical and mechanical safety device to avoid any accident
    - Should have low rotation speed for better gripping and cutting of waste

- Maximum rotation 50 rpm
- Discharge outlet should be at least 3 feet above ground to adjust the collection container for shredded waste
- Should have heavy motor to ensure efficient cutting of waste
- Should be designed to allow minimum manual handling.

55. **What is shredding?**

    Shredding is a process of waste treatment by which waste are deshaped or cut into smaller pieces so as to make the wastes unrecognizable. The process helps as a barrier in reuse of biomedical waste as well as acts as identifier that the wastes have been disinfected and are safe to dispose off.

56. **What should be precaution of storage at CBWTF?**

    There is need of two storeroom, one for treated waste and another for untreated waste and both should have smooth, fine surface which can be easily washed and has well ventilation. Floor should be impermeable to liquid.

57. **What difficulties are faced by CBWTF from health care institution?**
    - Health care facilities don't enroll themselves voluntarily to CBWTF.
    - Declaration of less number of beds
    - Irregular payments by hospitals and other health care institutions
    - Unsegregated waste given to the facility
    - Some institutions are located in very congested area where vehicle cannot enter
    - Waste is not being kept ready when vehicle comes leading to unnecessary delay
    - Bags are not properly tied leading to spillage of waste.

58. **What deficiencies may be encountered at incinerator?**
    - Unsegregated waste is incinerated
    - Power backup for incinerator is not available
    - Record keeping is not proper
    - Operation and maintenance of incinerator is not as per the laid down norm
    - Incinerator ash is not disposed off properly
    - Monitoring platform and porthole for stock is not proper.

59. **Which is a good measure for incinerator efficiency?**
    Carbon monoxide is a good measure because:
    - It is produced on incomplete combustion
    - Temperature of incinerator is less
    - Oxygen concentration is less than required.

60. **What are the financial aspects involved in proper BMWM?**
    - Provision of proper BMWM is mandatory under BMW (management and handling) Rules 1998
    - Avoidance of cost of accident and compensation due to streamlined process of BMWM
    - Financial facilities are available.

61. **What is the schedule for hospital waste incinerator monitoring?**
    Daily:
    - Checking of oxygen monitor
    - Cleaning of ash kit after each shift
    - Checking of operation of thermocouples
    - Checking of doors seals for proper fitting, air leakage or wear and tear
    - Check and clean under fire airports.

    Weekly:
    - Checking and cleaning of air blowers from debris
    - Lubrication of all latches and hinges
    - Checking and cleaning of burner flame rods.

    Fortnightly:
    - Check and cleaning of burners and any fuel leakage
    - Checking of control panels.

    Monthly:
    - Checking and cleaning of external surface of incinerator and stock
    - Repair of any minor wear and tear
    - Cleaning of both chambers from inside
    - Readjustment of burners if required.

    Six monthly:
    - Checking and painting of hot external surface
    - Check and paint equipment enamel if needed.

62. **What are the operational problems of incinerator?**
    - Excessive stock emission
    - Leakage of smoke

- Excessive consumption of fuel
- Incomplete burning of waste
- Black smoke from stack
- White smoke from stake.

63. **What are the reasons for excessive stake emission?**
    - Overcharging
    - Problem causing waste
    - Excessive infiltration of air from charging door
    - Temperature in secondary chamber is not adequately high
    - Inadequate air in secondary chamber
    - Excessive under fire air in primary chamber.

64. **What are the reasons for leakage of smoke from primary chamber?**
    - Excessive charging of primary chamber
    - Too high temperature of primary chamber
    - Excessive combustion air.

    This all lead to high positive pressure in primary chamber. The remedy for controlling the leakage is to:
    – Reduce the feed
    – Reduce the temperature
    – Adjust ash discharge from chamber to wet sump. A sump is a low space that collects any often—undesirable liquids such as water or chemicals.

65. **Give the reasons for excessive fuel consumption.**
    - Inconsistent charging of chamber
    - Leakage from door seal
    - Improper functioning of fuel burners
    - Improper primary chamber combustion air level and distribution.

66. **What are the reasons for incomplete burning of waste?**
    - Overcharging of the chamber
    - Too much wet waste charging
    - Malfunctioning of primary chamber
    - Insufficient under fire
    - Improper maintenance of the incinerator.

67. **Why sometimes there is black smoke emission from stake?**
    This indicates presence of unburned carbonaceous material which may be because of following reasons:
    - Incomplete combustion of waste
    - Overcharging of volatile material
    - Secondary chamber temperature is less

    The problem can be eliminated by rectifying these problems.

68. **What is the indication of white smoke from the stake?**
    This indicates that the presence of small aerosols in effluent gas. The white smoke is the result of finely divided non-combustible minerals present in the waste and this is being carried out of the stake. One of such minerals is calcium chloride.

69. **What are the causes of white smoke from stake?**
    - Temperature of secondary chamber is too low leading to premature cooling of combustion gases
    - Increased under fire air
    - Under used secondary burner.

    The problem of white smoke can be eliminated by removing the cause.

Chapter 11

Infection Control

1. **Why infection control is essential?**
   It is essential for well-being of patients and safety of both patients and staff of the institution. This is considered as quality standard of patient care.

2. **What are the modes of infection transmission?**
   The infection can be transmitted from patient to health care workers and vice versa. There are four main routes for infection transmission:
   1. **Blood borne:** Infected blood reaching to healthy blood through cuts, sharp injuries or through mucocutaneous and percutaneous route
   2. **Contact:** Hands contaminated from patients' infected body fluids, secretions, excretions or contaminated items coming in contact with mucous membrane or skin lesions. Very often large droplets from respiration tract contaminate the environment close to patient and infection is transmitted by contact of such infected secretion with mucous membrane or skin lesion.
   3. **Feco-oral route (drinking and eating):** Here the fecal flora of patients contaminate the water, hands or food thus spreading infection.
   4. **Air borne:** Inhalation of droplet nuclei are disposed in air.

3. **What is the principle of infectious disease transmission?**
   For an infectious disease to get transmitted following conditions are essential:
   To understand and appreciate issues concerning the handling and disposing of biomedical waste, the principles of disease transmission must be understood. The segregation of potentially

infectious waste from the bulk of the solid waste stream—all of which could theoretically be considered "potentially infectious material" is a difficult task. Thus a working knowledge of the way in which infectious agents grow, multiply, and actually induce infection is essential to the development of an effective set of policies.
- Sufficient load of infectious is essential to induce an infection.
- The infectious agents should be viable as growth of agents requires specific conditions related to temperature, light, nutrients, pH conditions and moisture.
- A portal of exit so that agents get out of one source.
- Movement of an infectious agent from a source to the appropriate portal of entry in a susceptible host or individual. There are four principal methods of disease transmission and these are physical contact with an infected person including their secretions, excretions, body fluids or tissues; through the air; through food and water; and by indirect contact through vectors or other objects.
- A portal of entry in the susceptible host so as to cause infection.
- A susceptible host and in the context of BMWM these susceptible hosts are waste handlers at any stage of the management process. In community level rag pickers can be the susceptible hosts.

4. What are the risk factors for acquiring infection?

    Environment: A highly contaminated environment of the health care setting or high risk procedures whether diagnostic or therapeutic.
    Patient: Malnutrition, suppressed immune system extremes of age, injuries.
    Microbes: Highly virulent organism, bacterial load and presence of new strain or new minerals (Fig. 11.1).

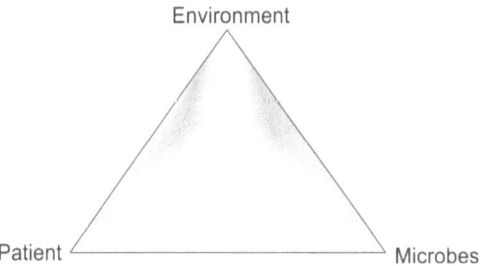

Fig. 11.1: Risk factors for infection.

5. **How the surveillance of infection is done?**
   Surveillance of the infection involves:
   - Collection of data on infection
   - Analysis of collected data
   - Feedback/recommendation to hospital staff

   Surveillance is mainly done in high risk areas like labor room, OT, laboratory, NICU, PICU, ICUS, etc. The data collected for surveillance are essential for developing and reviewing/revising infection control.

6. **What are the principles of infection control?**
   - Environment:
     - Designing of health care institution so as to have good ventilation
     - Meticulous cleaning
     - Positive pressure ventilation in high risk area
     - Effective BMW handling/treatment/disposal
     - Effective disinfections and sterilization of equipment.
   - Patients:
     - Admit those patients when absolute necessary
     - Barrier nursing for patients with depressed immunity
     - Provision of isolation ward for patients with communicable diseases
     - Hospital stay should be minimum possible
   - Microbes (agents)
     - Identification of the causative agent
     - Specific measures to prevent their spread.

7. **Which health care workers are at high risk of transmission of blood borne infection?**
   They are doctors, nurses, paramedical staff, lab technicians, housekeeping and laundry staff morticians.

8. **Which are the common organisms transmitted through blood/body fluids?**
   - Hepatitis B, C, virus
   - Cytomegalovirus
   - HIV
   - Epstein-Barr virus
   - Malaria parasites
   - Salmonella/Brucella.

9. **How much time does it take to deactivate HIV by boiling water?**
   HIV is deactivated by boiling water in seconds.

10. **What is the dose schedule for hepatitis B vaccination?**
    Hepatitis B vaccination is given in three doses. Second dose given one month after first dose and third dose given at 6 months after first dose. The dose schedule is 0 – 1 – 6.

11. **How passive immunization in hepatitis B is given?**
    Passive immunization is given with immunoglobulin and given with active immunization especially in case of proven accidental exposure to this infection in nonimmumized person. The dose is 0.06 mg per kg body weight and ideally be given within 72 hours of exposure.

12. **What is hepatitis C?**
    Hepatitis is single stranded RNA virus and it belongs to family of flaviviride. It is mainly transmited by blood and blood products. Sexual and perinatal transmission is also reported. The incubation period is 15 days to 24 weeks. The clinical features are malaise and jaundice. 50% may have cirrohosis or hepatocellular carcinoma. The virus is inactivated by wet heat and dry heat at 60°C and 80°C respectively. It can also be activated by chemicals like ether, chloroform, detergents and organic solvents.

13. **What is the most common way of blood borne infection?**
    Through accidental sharp injuries.

14. **What are the standard precautions in infection control?**
    - Barrier protection
    - Hand washing
    - Safe handling of sharps
    - Safe handling of spill of body fluid/blood
    - Meticulous housekeeping
    - Use of properly sterilized items
    - Use of safe techniques
    - Use of resuscitation bag or mouth piece instead of mouth-mouth resuscitation in case of emergency
    - Standardized laundry services
    - Regular medical checking.

15. **Where hand washing is mandatory?**
    - Before and after patients examination and patient care
    - Immediately after contact with blood/body fluids
    - Before handling food/drink/leaving the work place
    - After removing gloves/gown, etc.

16. **How the sharps be handled in health care setting?**
    - All chipped and broken glassware be discarded properly
    - Disposable needles should not be reapped, burnt, broken or removed from syringes
    - Dispose own sharp taking due care
    - Sharp container should be located near the generation point
    - Care taken not to get autoinoculated
    - Sharp container should be puncture proof and sent for disposal when three-fourth full
    - Use needle destroyer to mutilate sharp needle and present reuse
    - Used needles are disinfected with 5-1% hypochlorite solution or common bleach solution for 30 minutes
    - Used sharps should not be passed from one person to another person
    - Chemical disinfections should not be used as method of sterilization.

17. **What are the prerequisite for proper spill management?**
    The spill whether large or small should be managed properly taking care that staff does not get exposed to infected spilled material.
    - All staff members should be trained and educated in managing biomedical waste and recognizing and managing spill.
    - There should be laid down policy of managing spills.
    - Only designated and trained staff get involved in spill management.
    - Information about individual substances and their management should be made available to all staff members on a 24x7 basis.
    - Spill management kit and written standard operating procedure (SOP) kept ready for the use all time at designated place in facility and information about this be available with cleaning team.

- Procedures for proper disposal of waste is documented according to the facility's BMWM program.

18. **How the spill of blood/body fluids be handled effectively?**
    - Cover the spill with paper napkin/gauge piece/dry cloth pour disinfectant solution (1% hypochlorite freshly prepared leave it for 30 minutes with gleaned hand paper napkin/dry/guage piece is removed.
    - Wash area with detergent soap and water.
    - All used material is treated and disposed as infectious waste.

19. **What precautions should be taken while handling soiled linen?**
    - Soiled linen be handled minimum so as to prevent gross microbial contamination of air and staff handling linen
    - Solid linen be decontaminated with bleach before sending to laundry
    - Linen washed in hot water (more than 70°C) and detergent
    - Gloves must be worn while handling soiled linen.

20. **Who all are involved in infection control?**
    Infection control committee consists of:
    - HOD, Microbiology – Chairman
    - Infection control officer – Secretary
    - Infection control nurse
    - Medical superintendent
    - Nursing superintendent
    - Quality assurance officer
    - HOD of all major/minor clinical department.

21. **Why infection surveillance in hospital required?**
    This is done in order to:
    - Determine the incidence of endemic infection in different areas of hospital
    - Determine the effectiveness of day-to-day control measures
    - Recognize any change in incidence of infection
    - Desirability and recommending any specific measure to control infection in hospital.

22. **What are the functions of infections control committee?**
    - Review efficacy of control measures
    - Formulation of hospital policy to review the infection related problem

- To provide adequate isolation facilities
- To recommend policies for disinfections and sterilization
- Assigning appropriate role to all members of the committee
- Preparation of SOPs
- Developing mechanism for dissemination of information.

23. **What is the composition of infection control team (ICT)?**
    - Infection control officer (ICO)
    - Microbiologist (if he/she is not ICO)
    - Infection control nurse
    - Epidemiologist
    - Clinician interested in hospital acquired infection.

24. **Mention day-to-day function of infection control team.**
    - Surveillance (discovery and recording) of infection
    - Monitoring of carriers
    - Regular training of all staff members on infection control
    - Advice control measures and periodically check its efficacy
    - Prepare factsheet on available data related to infection
    - Outbreak management
    - Day-to-day momentary sterilization, disinfection processes
    - Report back to infection control committee.

25. **Which parameters are monitored by waste management officers?**
    - Amount of waste generated (category-wise) in each department each month and their daily segregation, transport and treatment.
    - Planning and calculation of financial aspect of health care waste management this includes direct cost of material used in management training cost, cost for centralized services, cost of operations and maintenance of on site treatment facilities.
    - Public health aspect of BMW and reporting of waste related injury.
    - Ensure compliance of BMWM system with National Legislation.
    - Training awareness and coordination and conduction of BMW training.
    - Liaison with central and state pollution control board.

26. **What is the role of department head in BMWM?**
    - Ensure that all staff members are aware of segregation process of waste and comply to the hospital policy on waste management.
    - Ensure key members are given periodic training on BMWM.
    - Continuously liaison with waste management officers to monitor working practices in their department.
    - Encourage medical and nursing staff to stick with standardized practices of BMWM.

27. **What are the causes of spillage of blood/body fluids?**
    - Breakage of container
    - Over filling
    - Leaking
    - Tipping over container
    - Dropping of/from container
    - Splashing.

28. **What should be contents of spill kit?**
    - Bucket
    - Adsorbent (saw dust, gauge piece, etc.)
    - Gloves
    - Face mask
    - Disposable bag
    - Disinfectant.

Chapter 12

Occupational Hazards and Universal Precaution

1. **What are the dangerous byproducts of Healthcare?**
   Radioactive wastes, mercury containing instruments and polyvinyl chloride (PVC) plastics. These are among the most environmentally sensitive byproducts of healthcare.

2. **What cleaning devices are used by waste handlers?**
   Brooms: The broom shall be a minimum of 1.2 m (120 cm) long, so that worker need not stoop to sweep. The diameter of the broom should be convenient to firm grip of broom. The brush of the broom shall be soft or hard depending on the type of flooring to be cleaned.

   Dustpans: The dustpans should be used to collect the dust from the sweeping operations. They may be either of plastic or enameled metal. They should not have ribs and should have smooth contours, so as to prevent dust from sticking to the surface. They should be washed with disinfectants and dried before every use.

   Vacuum cleaners: Domestic vacuum cleaners or industrial vacuum cleaners can be used depending on the size of the rooms to be cleaned.

   Mops: Mops with long handles. Mops can be made of either the cloth or rubber. The mop has to be periodically replaced depending on the wear and tear. The mechanical screw type of mop is convenient for squeezing out the water.

3. **Enumerate biomedical waste handling occupational hazards.**
   The hazards can be categorized in the following:

Accidents:
- Wounds form sharp objects
- Chemical burns—by contact of hazardous chemical mixed with general waste
- Poisoning—accidental contact with hazardous chemicals complacently mixed with general waste
- Burns—may be caused by methane explosion at landfills sites or occupational accidents at final waste disposal sites.

Infections:
- Skin and blood infections—direct contact of waste with skin area having breach in continuity of skin or mucous membrane.
- Respiratory and eye infections—exposure to infected dust
- Intestinal infections—transmitted by flies feeding on the waste which is managed indiscriminately.

Chronic diseases: Chronic respiratory diseases, various types of cancers due to constant and long-term exposure to hazardous compounds during complete waste management cycle especially at common treatment facility (incinerator operator).

4. **Which are the diseases caused by biomedical waste (BMW)?**
   - Tuberculosis
   - Dermatitis and skin infections, bliss
   - Hepatitis B, C
   - HIV
   - Tetanus
   - Diarrheal diseases
   - Pneumonia
   - Conjunctivitis
   - Typhoid.

5. **Who all can be affected by BMW?**
   - Doctors
   - Nurses
   - Paramedical staff
   - Waste handlers
   - General public.

6. **Which are the routes through which BMW can cause infection?**
   - Inhalation
   - Ingestion
   - Injury

- Absorption
- Contamination of wounds.

7. **How the waste handlers are affected by BMW?**
   They are mostly affected by:
   - Emission from incinerator
   - Sharp injury
   - Exposure to radioactive waste
   - Inhalation of toxic waste products.

8. **What safety measures be taken by staff handling BMW?**
   - Personal protection items:
     - Plastic apron
     - Heavy duty rubber gloves
     - Mask
     - Eye shield
     - Gum boots about 6" above ankle
     - Covering of all cuts, wounds and abrasions.
   - Immunization against tetanus and hepatitis B
   - Accident reporting
   - Adoption of universal precaution
   - Awareness about hazards of BMW.

9. **Give the details of personnel safety devices.**
   Gloves: Heavy-duty rubber gloves should be used by waste handlers. This should be bright yellow in color. After handling the waste, the gloves should be washed twice. The gloves should be washed after every use with carbolic soap and a disinfectant. The size of gloves should fit the user.
   Aprons/gown: This should be worn to prevent contamination of clothing and protect skin. It should be made of impermeable material, such as plastic. Staff working in incinerator chambers should have gowns or suits made of noninflammable material.
   Masks: Various types of masks, goggles, and face shields are worn alone or in combination to provide a protective barrier. It is mandatory for staff working in the incinerator chamber to wear a mask covering both nose and mouth, preferably a gas mask with filters.
   Boots: Leg coverings, boots provide protection to the skin when splashes or large quantities of infected waste have to be handled. The boots should be rubber sole and antiskid type. They should cover the leg above ankle.

10. **What are the determinant factors for occupational exposure of HIV?**
    - Number of exposures
    - Type of exposures, i.e. percutaneous, mucosal, cutaneous
    - Type of body fluid—blood, body fluid
    - Viral load at time of exposure
    - Fresh or old fluid at the time of exposure.

11. **On what factors does the severity of injury depend?**
    - Depth of injury
    - Duration of contact
    - Hollow or solid needle
    - Size of wound
    - Bore size of needle
    - Vascularity of area of injury
    - Amount of blood/fluid injected.

12. **What factors are preventive for a healthcare worker?**
    - Healthy immunological status
    - Protective precautions while working
    - Attentive and careful worker
    - Methodological working sticking to standard operating procedures (SOPs) for particular task/process
    - Availability of first aid and postexposure prophylaxis (PEP) in case of exposure.

13. **Why are universal precautions essential?**
    - Any percutaneous or permucosal exposure to blood or body fluids which may be potential source
    - It is a part of patient care strategy to prevent discrimination against HIV injected patients and non-HIV
    - If healthcare workers feel that they can protect themselves from dreaded infections then they provide better care.

14. **What are the components of universal precautions?**
    - **Precautions for exposure to blood and body fluids:**
        - Personal protective equipment
        - Engineering control
        - Work practice control.
    - Ensure universal precaution
    - Behavior modification
    - Ensure adherence to universal precautions
    - Implications to surgeons.

15. **Who is responsible for preventing occupational hazards?**
    It is the prime responsibility of employer by following the under mentioned procedures:
    - Proactive action to prepare guidelines to avoid occupational hazards
    - Creating awareness among healthcare workers
    - Training and retraining about safe BMWM.
16. **What are downstream risks?**
    These are the risks related to biomedical waste beyond the healthcare settings. The causes may be:
    - Accidental contact with pathogen or toxic material
    - Discarded pharmaceutical products
    - Used but intact medical devices like blood set, syringes, blades, etc.
17. **Which heavy metals are common in BM waste?**
    - Mercury
    - Nickel
    - Cadmium
    - Copper
    - Chromium
    - Lead.
18. **What are most common occupational health hazards related to BM waste?**
    - Respiratory tract problems
    - Needle stick injuries
    - Lead poisoning from the burning of material containing lead
    - Back and joint injury due to lifting heavy waste loads
    - Nausea and headache due to unhygienic waste dump site and obnoxious smell
    - Infections.
19. **What is the role of counseling in prevention of occupational hazards?**
    Counseling allows staff and workers to receive individually targeted information about the risk related to waste and preventive aspects and methods of occupationally acquired infections.
20. **How the occupational hazards are classified?**
    - Physical
    - Biological
    - Chemical

- Psychological
- Ergonomic.

21. **What is ergonomics?**
    It is concerned with the factors that come into interplay when work is adopted to the worker.
22. **What are usual ergonomic hazards?**
    - Incorrect postures
    - Wrong equipments and tools
    - Bad design of workplace.
23. **Which organs are most vulnerable to microwave radiations?**
    Cornea and lens because of absence of heat dissipating blood vessels.
24. **What are the employers responsibilities to prevent occupational health hazards?**
    - Provision of safe workplace complying with all standards, rules and regulations
    - Periodic examination of the workplace to ensure compliance to standards
    - Liberal use of posters, signs, labels to aware employees constantly about occupational hazards
    - Regular and proper maintenance of equipment and tools and machines
    - Preparation of guidelines and SOPs
    - Regular medical examination of staff exposed to hazards
    - Training as and when required.
25. **When the health surveillance of an employee be done?**
    - Health assessment before staff is appointed on the job
    - During employment there will be periodic medical examinations of an employed
    - Health assessment of employee when they are returning after long leave
    - At the time of retirement, release, termination and resignation.
26. **How occupational safety in healthcare institution be established?**
    By developing following health and safety program in the institution:
    - Identification of hazards by regular record check and personal observations
    - Evaluation of hazard by regular waste evaluation program

- Training of employees and all other concerned staff
- Implementation of appropriate control measures
- Maintenance of all surveys related records meticulously
- Top management support for implication of program
- Financial supports to safety programs.

27. **What is the meaning of PEP?**
    Post-exposure prophylaxis is most useful in case of HIV and hepatitis B infection.

28. **What are the immediate steps to be taken in case of exposure?**
    - Wash the needle stick or cut area with soap and plenty of water
    - Irrigate eye with water or saline
    - Mucous membrane splash to be flushed with water
    - Never put pricked finger in mouth reflexly.

29. **Which forms are used for accident reporting and needle stick injury?**
    - Accident injury form no. 1
    - Needle stick injury form no. 2.

30. **What percentage of inhaled mercury fumes are absorbed in the body?**
    About 75-85% of dose is absorbed.

31. **What is the seroconversion rate for HBV, HCV and HIV due to biomedical waste?**
    It is 30%, 3% and 0.3%, respectively for HBV, HCV and HIV.

32. **Who is the healthcare worker?**
    Any person whose activities involve contact with patients or patients' blood or body fluids in a health care or laboratory setting.

33. **What steps are taken on exposure to HIV infected blood or body fluids and contaminated sharp?**
    - Immediate action:
        - Washing of injured or splash area with soap and water
        - Eye should be irrigated with plenty of water or saline
        - Do not put pricked finger in mouth.
    - Exposure incident reported to appropriate authority in the institution.
    - Post-exposure prophylaxis (PEP) given based on:
        - Degree of exposure to HIV
        - HIV status of the source.

- PEP as per the protocol
- HIV testing and counseling
- PEP should be started as early as possible because after 72 hours it is of no use and not recommended and once started the therapy should continue for 4 weeks
- If HIV testing is found to be positive within 12 weeks then HCW should be referred to physicians for treatment.

34. **What is the schedule for HIV testing in case of exposure?**
    Baseline HIV testing – at time of exposure
    Repeat HIV test – 6 weeks after exposure
    Second repeat HIV test – 12 weeks after exposure.

35. **What precautions should be taken by HCW during this period?**
    - Abstain from sexual intercourse
    - Refrain from donation of blood, semen, organ or tissue
    - Surgeon refrain from doing surgery
    - Females not to breastfeed their babies.

36. **What is exposure code?**
    It is the code given to the degree exposure in severity based on exposure, intactness of skin and/or mucous membrane and volume of the body fluid/blood.

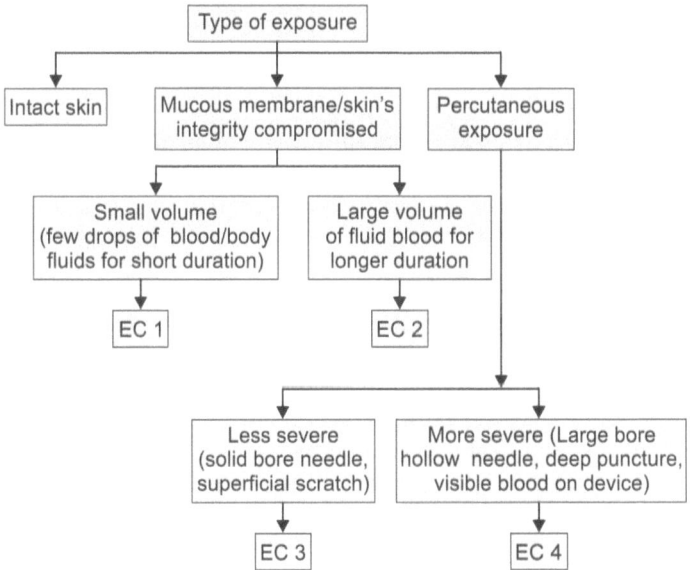

37. How HIV status of source is determined?
With the help of following flowchart.

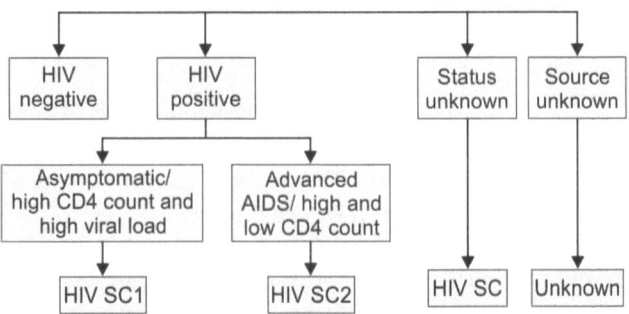

38. What are PEP recommendations based on expose code (EC) and HIV status code (SC)?

EC	HIV SC	PEP recommendation
1	1	No PEP warranted
1	2	Consider basic regimen
2	1	Recommend basic regimen
2	2	Recommend expanded regimen
3	1 or 2	Recommend expanded regimen
2 or 3	Unknown	Consider basic regimen

39. Which drugs are used in basic regimen and expanded regimen?

Basic regimen: Zidovudin 600 mg is divided dose plus lamivudin 150 g twice a day for 4 weeks

Expanded regimen: Basic regimen plus Indinavir 800 g three times a day for 4 weeks.

40. What is bloodborne pathogen exposure control plan?

This is the written document which identify the task and procedures as well as job description where there are chances of occupational exposure to blood occurs. The plan gives details about provision of standards and specify the procedures for the purpose of evaluating circumstances surrounding exposure incidents. All staff member should be able to access the plan and management should review the plan and update at least annually however changes can be brought anytime if necessity arises to do so.

41. **What are the reasons which make hepatitis B infection very serious?**
    The seriousness about hepatitis B infection is because of two reasons:
    1. The virus is very durable as it can survive in dried blood for up to 7 days hence it is of primary concern for the hospital staff like laundryman, waste handlers, CSSD staff, etc.
    2. There is no specific treatment or cure for hepatitis B however those who get infected will develop antibodies in their blood against this virus antigen which will help them to get over the infection and protect them from reinfection. However, these individuals who are having antibodies against hepatitis B are not immune to other forms of hepatitis.

42. **What are the symptoms of hepatitis B infection ?**
    The initial symptoms are very much similar to "flu" like including body fatigue, anorexia, stomach ache, and even retching sensation. As the infection continues to develop the person will have jaundice and dark urine. The incubation period is 1-9 months but anorexia and stomach ache may occur as early as with 1-3 months (2 weeks) or may get delayed till 6-9 months after infection.

43. **What is the dose schedule for hepatitis B vaccination?**
    Hepatitis B vaccination is given in three doses. Second dose given 1 month after first dose and third dose given at 6 months after first dose. The dose schedule is 0 - 1 - 6.

44. **How passive immunization in hepatitis B is given?**
    Passive immunization is given with immunoglobulin and given with active immunization especially in case of proven accidental exposure to this infection in non-immumized person. The dose is 0.06 mg per kg body weight and ideally be given within 72 hours of exposure.

45. **What is hepatitis C?**
    Hepatitis is single stranded RNA virus and it belongs to family of flaviviride. It is mainly transmited by blood and blood products. Sexual and perinatal transmission is also reported. The incubation period is 15 days to 24 weeks. The clinical features are malaise and jaundice. 50% may have cirrohosis or hepatocellular carcinoma. The virus is inactivated by wet heat and dry heat at 60°C and 80°C respectively. It can also be activated by chemicals like ether, chloroform, detergents and organic solvents.

156   Occupational Hazards and Universal Precaution

46. **What is the protocol for gloves to prevent occupational exposure?**
    - Gloves must be disposable
    - Change gloves after one hour. Total time a gloves can be used is 3 hours
    - In high-risk patient care double gloves must be used
    - In routine single glove is sufficient
    - Wash hand thoroughly with soap before wearing gloves and after degloving
    - Do not touch the area which is not involved in diagnostic or treatment procedures
    - Cover the cuts/wounds on hand with waterproof bandaid before putting on gloves
    - Check the gloves for any defect before putting them on
    - Discard gloves at the least suspicious of puncture.

47. **What is the protocol for mask wearing?**
    - Mask preferably should be disposable
    - Mask should be of good fitting
    - Mask should be discharged after any surgical procedure which is lasting more than 20 minutes or where aerosol spray expected or surgical procedure on high-risk patient
    - Mask should be disinfected with liquid bleach before washing.

48. **From occupational safety point of view what precautions should be taken by hospital staff dealing with BMW?**
    Following are the staff safety provisions while handling BMW:
    - All the staff who are involved in handling of biomedical waste (BMW) should be immunized against hepatitis B and tetanus to certain high-risk workers dealing with waste.
    - BMW should not be touched with bare hands.
    - Never recap used syringes.
    - Do not mix general waste and BMW at any given point of time from segregation to disposal.
    - Contaminated, damaged or poorly maintained PPE should not be used.
    - Good quality PPE should be used while handling BMW and these PPE should be replace periodically.
    - Intermediate storage room should be kept neat and clean. It should be senitized regularly.
    - BMW segregation process should be monitored closely and use of appropriate color coded bags for collection is ensured.

Chapter 13

Mercury Waste Management

1. **Which metal is in liquid form at room temperature?**
   Mercury is the only metal which is liquid at room temperature.

2. **What is the one natural source for mercury emissions in the atmosphere?**
   Volcanoes.

3. **Why mercury is called global contaminant?**
   Mercury is called global contaminant because it is transported to long distances on air currents and then get deposited from atmosphere. This metal is known to get accumulated in body cells of living organisms thus pose health risks.

4. **What are ways in the healthcare facility through which the mercury emitted in the atmosphere?**
   The use of mercury-containing items in every healthcare facility gives rise to many ways for mercury emission and few of these important are:
   - Hospital waste incinerators where the biomedical waste mixed with waste containing mercury is burnt.
   - Release of mercury in to the waste water streams in and around healthcare facility.
   - Without pretreatment the mercury admixed waste is landfilled.
   - Mercury spillage in wards/departments.

5. **Why mercury is considered most toxic metal of hospital waste?**
   Because mercury is easily vaporized and may remain in atmosphere for long period causing long-term adverse effects.

Mercury Waste Management

6. **How mercury causes its adverse effects?**
   Through the inhalation of mercury vapors which is due to spill of mercury and which is not cleared properly.

7. **How the mercury produces its effects?**
   It gets absorbed in the body because of lipid solubility though metallic mercury is not rapidly absorbed. However, absorption of methyl mercury is virtually total, i.e. 90-95%. If mercury vapors are inhaled these vapors easily cross alveolar membrane and enter the bloodstream.

8. **Which instrument/equipment in hospital contains mercury?**
   - Sphygmomanometer
   - Thermometer
   - Ryle's tube
   - Dilators
   - Laboratory reagents.

9. **How the mercury spill is handled?**
   - Area specified where spill has occurred with the help of colored chalk
   - Open all windows and door to the outside
   - Wear gloves, mask and apron
   - Syringe containing water is used to suck the mercury
   - Mercury collected in glass container which is sealed
   - Area of spill is thoroughly cleaned with detergent and water.

10. **What is amount of mercury in BP apparatus and thermometer?**
    BP apparatus 60 g/BP apparatus
    Thermometer 0.61 g/thermometer

11. **Which is most hazardous to human body?**
    Methyl mercury is most toxic to human body and it is formed due to chemical modification of elemental mercury to methyl mercury. It affects CNS, lungs, skin, eyes, and kidneys.

12. **What should never be done in case of mercury spill?**
    - Never use vacuum cleaner to clean mercury because vacuuming will put mercury into air and increase exposure
    - Don't touch the mercury with bare hands
    - Never pour mercury into drain
    - Never use broom to clean mercury because it will break it into small droplets which can be easily inhaled

- Never wash soiled cloth in washing machine as latter may get contaminated and water from it may further contaminate sewer
- Never walk around with the shoes which are contaminated with mercury spills
- Remove all jewelry while handling mercury because it reacts with mercury.

13. **What do you understand by "phasing out mercury" in the hospital?**

    It is the process of replacement of mercury containing equipment by non-mercury equipment. Many hospitals have phased out thermometer and sphygmomanometer under this program.

14. **How "phasing out mercury" is achieved in hospital?**

    By observing following practices:
    - Recycling of mercury containing product
    - Proper management of mercury spills
    - Use of alternative mercury free products
    - Proper management of mercury and mercury containing equipments
    - Waste management practices which reduce the discharge of mercury into environment.

15. **What are the advantages of mercury pollution precaution?**
    - Reduction in occupational exposure
    - Cost contaminant in recycling and tackling hazards related to mercury pollution
    - Increased awareness of community population.

16. **Why the mercury removal from the healthcare facility is advantageous?**

    It is because of under mentioned reasons:
    - 99% of mercury in healthcare facility is contained in esophageal dilators, sphygmomanometer, thermometer and service kits
    - The risk of mercury spillage is very high and the cost of spillage management is also equally high
    - The cost of mercury replacement is modest in comparison to cost of spillage management. Hence mercury items should be replace with non mercury items. Example replacement of mercury containing thermometer to digital thermometer

- Removal of mercury from hospital means "get out of the hospital" not mere out of services
- Purchase department should be vigilant that not mercury should enter the facility training on mercury audit should be done on one to one basis as in large group it would lose the impact and will not be successful.

17. **What about mercury control in healthcare facilities?**
    Every healthcare facility produces solid waste which contain variable quantity of mercury. The source of mercury may be due to breakage of sphygmomanometer, thermometer, etc. The mercury waste management is not concerned with it final disposal but also with collection of spilled mercury, its storage and sending back to product manufacturer. Also due care to be taken that mercury waste does not become part of either biomedical or general waste. As mentioned in Schedule – 2 of Hazardous Waste (management and handling) Rules, 2003, any waste containing equal to or more than 50 ppm of mercury is hazardous waste and concerned generator of such waste, whether healthcare or nonhealthcare facility, require to follow the Hazardous Waste **(HW)** Rules to dispose of these waste.

18. **How much quantity of mercury a clinical thermometer contains?**
    The quantity of mercury in clinical thermometer varies from 0.5 g to 3.0 g.

19. **What are the main reason for thermometer breakage in clinical practice?**
    The usual way a thermometer gets broken is due to slipping from hands while it is being shaken to bring the temperature down.

20. **What is the average number of breakage of thermometer per month in clinical practice?**
    It is estimated that average monthly breakage is around 70 per month in 300 bedded nonteaching hospital. In case of teaching hospital the number will further increase.

21. **What is dental amalgam?**
    It the mercury alloy which is primarily used in dental practice to do dental filling.

22. **What is amalgam tattoo?**
    After amalgam filling the mercury from it starts getting free either by external mechanical/biological influences or by vaporization and gets impregnated in the surrounding gums. After few years in some patients this impregnated mercury develops a silvery line on gums and this is called amalgam tattoo.

23. **What are the nonmercury options available in dental practice?**
    These are as follows:
    - Glass ionomer cement
    - Gold foil
    - Gold alloy
    - Ceramic fillings

24. **How much quantity of mercury a dentist must be using on annual basis?**
    It is around 1 kg to 1.5 kg.

    What is esophageal dilator (bougie)?
    It is the long, flexible tube made of this latex and used for dilating esophageal strictures.

25. **Where is the mercury in esophageal bougie?**
    It is at the bottom of the bougie.

26. **What is the purpose of keeping mercury at the bottom of bougie?**
    The main purpose is to use it as weight at the bottom so that the tube can easily slip down due to its weight. Secondly due to liquid property of mercury it is ideal flexible weight so that it does not cause harm to the esophageal tissues.

27. **What are the areas in hospital where mercury is used?**
    - Dental department
    - Endoscopy room
    - Pathology laboratory
    - Pharmacy
    - Stores
    - Emergency department
    - Outpatient department (OPD)
    - Biomedical equipment department

28. **What happens once mercury enters in to the environment?**
   Once mercury enters in to environment it remains there permanently because of its persistent and bioaccumulative property it never breakdown into harmless or inert form. It also keep changing its chemical form which depending on environment.

29. **Why mercury remain so popular in medical practice?**
   The choice of mercury remain on the top because of its unique combination of weight, high boiling point, chemical stability, ability to flow, electrical conductivity, and relatively low vapor pressure.

30. **What are the physical properties of mercury?**
   Elemental mercury is heavy, liquid as room temperature, melthing and boiling points are 38.90 and 357°C. Due to high surface tension the drops appears to be round in shape. The density at 25 °C is 13.5 g/cm^3.

31. **Name the few metals with which mercury can get combined.**
   Gold, silver, copper and tin. The combination is known as amalgams (alloys).

32. **Which is the metal with which mercury does not combine?**
   The metal is iron which does not combine with mercury.

33. **What happens when mercury is evaporates?**
   On evaporation it forms colorless and odorless gas.

34. **Why mercury spreads to larger area when it spills?**
   On spilling mercury breaks in to very small droplets which due to high surface tension becomes rounds and hence rolls down to distant place from the point of spill.

35. **What is the role of room ventilation in mercury spill effects?**
   The proper room ventilation dilute the concentration of mercury in the confined atmosphere.

36. **On what factors the mercury vapor production depends?**
   The following factors are important
   - The volume of mercury spill
   - Room temperature (higher the temperature more the vapors)
   - Speed of air flow

- Handling of spilled mercury
- Total surface area of spilled mercury.

37. **What are the other factors which make essential of mercury spilled management?**
    These are because the spilled droplets can get:
    - Lodged in to floor cracks
    - Adhere to carpet or floor fabrics
    - Stick to shoe soles
    - Dissolved with other metals in rings, bangles and watches to form alloys/amalgams
    - Mix with dust
    - Mixed with drainage water and then goes to main stream.

38. **How healthcare professional can get exposed to mercury?**
    There are two routes through with any healthcare profession can get exposed to mercury:
    1. Inhalation of inorganic mercury vapor after spill because the spilled mercury increase the concentration in the air of that particular place
    2. Accidental skin contact with mercury.

39. **Why mercury spill in carpeted patient's room becomes a big challenge?**
    Because the spilled mercury get breakdown in to very tiny droplets and get fixed with carpet fabric.

40. **What are the impacts if mercury waste is not managed properly?**
    The unmanaged waste may get accessed to the ground water and then in to food chain thus affecting the environment and community at large scale. For this reason it is prudent to follow the 4 R principles which consists of Reuse, Recycle, Reduce, Recovery. Healthcare facility should try to eliminate use of mercury in the organization in phased manner.

41. **Which type of toxic effects mercury produces on body?**
    Mercury is a potent neurotoxic hence long time exposure affects peripheral as well as central nervous system (brain, spinal cord).

42. **What other organs get affected by mercury?**
    - Kidney
    - Liver

- Eyes
- Placenta through which affect the unborn child.

43. **How a person can get exposed to mercury?**
    There are three ways a person can get exposed to mercury:
    - Inhalation (most common)
    - Ingestion
    - Skin contacts.

44. **What are the clinical features of acute inhalation of mercury on body**
    Coughing, breathlessness, chest pain, anorexia, nausea, chills, increased salivation, gingivitis, diarrhea, gastroenteritis, nephritis, uremia, anuria, ataxia.

45. **What are the clinical features of chronic exposure to mercury on body?**
    Weakness, weight loss, gastrointestinal disturbances, tremor starting from fingers, eyelids, and lips and progressing to generalized seizures and violent spasms of the extremities. The affected person may have behavioral and personality changes which include increased excitability, amnesia, insomnia, and depression. In addition, there may be a painful scaling or peeling of the skin of the hands and feet.

46. **What are the strategies a healthcare facility should adapt while managing waste containing mercury?**
    A healthcare facility should adapt the following strategies while managing mercury containing waste:
    - Established policy and standard operating procedures (SOPs) for mercury management
    - Proper segregation of waste
    - Recycling of mercury containing waste
    - Careful handling of mercury containing equipments
    - Carefully managing mercury spillage
    - Regular monitoring of compliance to mercury management policies
    - In phased manner changing over to nonmercury products.

47. **What are the mercury free alternatives for hospitals?**
    Mercury free alternatives are as follows:
    - Aneroid and electronic BP machines

- Replacing mercury bougie by Tungsten get bougie
- Nonmercury amalgams
- Electronic thermometer
- Use of zinc chloride based fixatives in laboratory.

48. **How mercury containing instruments be stored?**
    Following guidelines should be used to store mercury containing instruments:
    - The container should not have hard bottom
    - Plastic containers are preferred because of their softness
    - The cleaning should be done at designated place and by trained staff only
    - The calibration should be done while keeping instrument in the stray so any spill occur remains limited to tray only
    - Instruments should not be used in carpeted rooms
    - Instruments should not be used in the place where there are high projected portions of patient bed or in the area where patient cannot be moved quickly in case of spill.

49. **What action should be taken in case of mercury spill due to mercury containing instrument breakage?**
    Following guidelines will be useful in case there is instrument breakage and mercury spill:
    - Remove patients and staff from the spill area
    - Minimize vaporization of spilled mercury by switching off heaters
    - Switch off ACs so as to reduce the circulation of mercury vapors to other sensitive areas
    - Maintain proper ventilation by opening windows and ventilators
    - Manage the spill immediately by trained staff irrespective of spill amount
    - Staff who manages spill should use personal protective equipment (PPE)
    - After spill management hands should be washed thoroughly
    - All the articles used in spill management should be kept separately and stored in designated area
    - Rinse the area thoroughly and dry mop.

Below mentioned practices should not be followed while handling mercury spill:
- Vacuum cleaner not to be used because it will contaminate vacuum cleaner and heat from cleaner will vaporize mercury thus increasing exposure
- Spilled mercury should not be handled with bare hands
- While doing spill management jewelry should be removed
- Broom should not be used to clean mercury spill because it further breaks mercury in to tiny droplets which are hard to collect and spread to larger areas
- Mercury waste should not be discharged in to common drainage
- Mercury soiled linens not be washed in washing machine as this will contaminate the general sewage system
- Mercury soiled items should not be burned in open to avoid mercury into atmosphere.

50. **What are the items kept in mercury spill management kit?**
The kit should contain—once the items in the kit are used them they should be immediately be replaced. This responsibility is headed by the spill management team leader.

51. **How one should ensure that the items used have been replaced?**
The kit should have a sheet which has the details when the kit was use by whom and kit replenished by whom. The sheet should be dated and signed by designated staff.

Mercury spill management kit

Date	Place of spill	Type of spill (major/minor)	Kit used by (name)	Signature	Kit items replenished by (name)	Signature

52. **Where should be these kits be kept?**
The mercury spill management kits should be kept at the places where they can be accessed by the staff immediately in case of spill occurs. The information about the kit should be available to all the trained staff members.

53. **What are the steps in mercury spill management?**
   Following steps should be followed to manage spill successfully:
   - Ask everyone to leave the area of spill
   - Area of spill is cordoned
   - Ventilation system turned off
   - Spill handling team remove jewelry then put on old cloths and PPE
   - Mercury beads are located.

54. **How the mercury waste is stored?**
   The waste is stored in designated storage areas which has following facilities:
   - Air conditioned to prevent the vaporization of mercury
   - Sufficient light
   - Smooth surface by epoxy
   - Mercury spill management kit.

55. **What is the maximum period a healthcare facility can keep mercury waste before transporting it for final disposal?**
   According to Hazardous Waste (Management, Handling and Transboundary Movement) Rules, 2008 notified under Environment Protection Act, 1986, in consultation with respective SPCB the maximum period the mercury waste can be kept is 90 days.

56. **What precautions should be taken while storing mercury waste?**
   Below mentioned precautions needs to be considered while storing mercury waste:
   - The area should be designated with locking facility or incase it partitioned then that area should not be used very frequently
   - The storage area should bear the signage
   - Waste should be stored away from the sensitive sites, e.g. school, residential area, food industry, agricultural land, healthcare facility, etc.
   - The container should be of metal or hard plastic and should be in good condition
   - The drainage of the storage site should be away from it
   - The floor of storage should be made either of concrete to which epoxy covering done or should have durable plastic sheet of 6 mm thickness

- Audit system of storing conditions (leaks, fire alarms, vandalism, degradation of container materials, sprinklers, etc.) be in place and this should be in the format of date, observation of auditor, name and signature
- Containers to be handled by trained staff only
- A copy of material safety data sheet (MSDS) should be made available in the storage area
- The waste should be transported by authorized transporter only.

57. **What are other options of mercury waste management?**
    Available other options are:
    - Waste pickup and disposal by equipment manufacturer under the scheme of extended producer responsibility (EPR)
    - Disposal of mercury waste through mercury recovery units
    - Disposal through hazardous waste treatment, storage and disposal facility (TSDF)
    - Disposal through common biomedial waste treatment facility (CBWTF).

58. **What is the best way to monitor the mercury in healthcare facility?**
    The facility should maintain and update all records related to mercury in the form of instruments, equipments, purchase, broken, in use etc. It is advisable also that facility maintain up to date record of spills management as well including place of spill, collection, storage and final disposal. The annual report needs to be submitted according to biomedical waste (management and handling) Rules, 1998. The deadline for annual report submission is on or before 31st January every year.

59. **How awareness about mercury waste management can be brought among the staff members?**
    A besides periodic training the other methods are:
    - Workshops
    - Seminar
    - Display of posters at strategic location across the facility
    - Computer based in the form of screen saver or wallpaper
    - Notices and placards.

60. **In what way exposure to mercury vapor be reduced at the time of spill management?**
    The spill managed by trained staff in the shortest possible time.

61. **What are the mode of mercury release in environment from mercury based equipments?**
    As the details given here:

Sr No	Instrument/equipment	Mode of mercury release
1	Thermometer	Slipping from hand and breakage
2	BP instrument	Slipping and breakage during use
3	Dental amalgam	Mercury get released from amalgam and form amalgam tattoo
4	Esophageal bougie	Leak or breakage
5	Feeding tube	Leak or breakage
6	Urinometer	Breakage
7	X-ray machine	Release due to improper handling
8	Batteries	Breakage
9	Laboratory chemicals	Drain in to sewage system

62. **What are the features of good biomedical waste management system in an institution?**
    The following are the essential requirements for medical waste management:
    - Laid down policies and SOPs
    - Development of waste management plan along with contingency plan
    - Allocation of resources financial as well as human resource
    - Implementation of plan and action
    - Proper monitoring and evaluation
    - Periodic training of concerned staff
    - Endeavor to have continuous improvements
    - Environmental preferable purchasing (EPP), i.e. purchase of product which are environmentally sound and friendly.

63. **What the meaning of satellite in the field of BMWM?**
    It is the location near or at the point of biomedical waste generation. At this place the waste is initially accumulated in containers and then consolidated.

64. **What are the effects of mercury waste on lake water?**
    Once the mercury is discharged in to the lake water by any means it gets accumulated in lake bottom sediments and get transformed in to more toxic organic form called methyl mercury.

This methyl mercury accumulates in the body tissue of fish thus ultimately affect human health adversely.

65. **What percentage of inhaled mercury gets absorbed in to the blood?**
   About 80% gets absorbed in to the blood.

66. **What is the composition of dental amalgam?**
   It contains 45-50% mercury and around 30% is silver and other metals such as copper, zinc and tin, etc.

67. **According to WHO what is the nonindustrial source of mercury exposures?**
   Dental amalgam is the greatest source of mercury exposure.

68. **What is the occupational exposure of mercury?**
   It is via inhalation of liquid mercury vapors. The mercury spillage if not managed properly may lead to higher concentration of mercury in indoor air above the recommended level.

69. **What are the strategies of mercury free healthcare?**
   WHO has brought forward short-term, medium as well as long-term strategies to tackle mercury menace.
   Short-term strategy—it consists of following components:
   - Laid down mercury spill and waste management protocols
   - Periodic mock drill, training and education to all concerned staff members
   - Slowly replace mercury containing equipment by nonmercury containing equipments.

   Medium-term strategy—below mentioned action plan is part of medium-term strategy:
   - Reduce the number of mercury containing equipments
   - Healthcare organization should maintain the mercury use inventory which should have been classified in to two subgroups one immediately replaceable and another slowly replaceable.
   - The plan should be in place that while getting rid of mercury containing equipments these should be taken back by manufacturer or alternative equipment providers.
   - Organization should ensure that returned mercury equipments are not place back in to supply chain.

Long-term strategy—it consists of the following steps:
- Every healthcare organization should support the ban on use of mercury containing devices.
- Organization should prepare and keep in place a very sound action plan for mercury containing waste management.
- Allocate sufficient resources to manage mercury containing waste properly.

70. **What is the popular norm in regards to mercury use?**
Pollution prevention is much better, faster and cheaper than pollution control.

Chapter 14

Management of Specialized Waste

1. **What are the specialized wastes in hospital?**
   - Heavy metals like lead, cadmium, mercury
   - Radiological waste
   - Radioactive waste
   - Pharmaceutical waste
   - Cytotoxic waste
   - Pressurized containers.

2. **Why are they called specialized waste?**
   Because their management process is different from the general process and each special waste needs individualized treatment, storage and disposal option.

3. **How cytotoxic waste is disposed?**
   It is disposed in one of the following manners:
   - Incineration at very high temperature (more than 120°C)
   - Return to original supplier
   - Chemical degradation so that it turns into nontoxic compounds
   - Inertization and encapsulation.

4. **Which methods are utilized for chemical degradation of cytotoxic waste?**
   Sulfuric acid or potassium per magnate for oxidation process, while hydrobromic acid for denitrosation.

5. **How pressurized containers are managed?**
   Undamaged containers returned to suppliers for reuse or recycle while damaged containers are crushed and disposed in secured landfills.

Management of Specialized Waste

6. **What precautions should be taken during segregation of pressurized containers?**
   These should not be placed in yellow container or bag which goes for incineration because on burning of sealed container there is a risk of explosion.

7. **Give treatment and disposal action for pharmaceutical waste.**
   There are different options for such waste depending on the quantity:

Small quantity	Large quantity
• Encapsulation	• Encapsulation
• Landfill	• Incineration at high temperature
• Dilution and discharge in sewer slowly (not for antibiotics and cytotoxic waste)	• Returned to original suppliers
• Safe burial	
• If less than 1% of total waste then incineration at high temperature (>1200°C)	

8. **How the sealed vials and ampoules be managed?**
   These are crushed on hard surface and with help of sieve medicine and glass are separated. The medicine is treated by inertization or encapsulation and glass is treated and disposed as sharp waste.

9. **How is radioactive waste managed?**
   It is managed as per the guidelines provided by BARC and atomic energy regulatory body.

10. **How many types of radioactive waste are there?**
    These are of 3 types:
    1. Radioactive solid waste
    2. Radioactive liquid waste
    3. Radioactive gaseous waste.

11. **What is radioactive waste?**
    It is the waste type containing radioactive elements that do not have a practical purpose hence need to be treated and disposed to avoid exposure and health problem related to radioactive waste.

12. **What is ionizing radiation?**
    It is the radiation which has the power to penetrate the tissue and infuse the energy into them leading to death of tissue.

13. **How radioactive waste causes contamination of human body?**
    It contaminates the human body through:
    - Ingestion
    - Inhalation
    - Injection
    - Absorption.

14. **What is effluent?**
    It is an outflowing of water from the hospital's various departments. It is considered highly pollutant.

15. **How many types of radioactive waste are there?**
    - **Low level waste:** Has short lived radioactivity, dormant, needs shielding during handling and transport and is suitable for shallow land burial. This type of waste is generated by hospitals
    - **Intermediate level waste:** Contains higher amounts of radioactivity, may need shielding, disposed off after encapsulation disposed in deep underground
    - **High level waste:** Very high level of radioactivity arises in nuclear reactors.

    Majority of radioactive wastes are low level waste.

16. **What is radioactive decay?**
    This is the process of continuous spontaneous disintegration of radioactive material. During decay radioactive material keeps emitting ionizing radiation either alfa, beta or gamma rays.

17. **How radioactive waste are disposed?**
    Low activity waste: Can be discharged into sewer where disposal occurs by dilution

    High activity waste: Subjected to pretreatment before disposal. Radionucleids are separated by ion exchange, precipitation or coagulation and then disposed of safely by burial

    Very high activity waste: Have to be stored indefinitely. They are stored in concrete filled steel drum and placed in the sea at the depth of 6,000 feet for all time.

18. **What does this sign indicate?**
    This is biohazard sign.

19. **How is liquid chemical waste from hospital managed?**
    The liquid chemical waste is fresh neutralized with reagent (acidic to basic and vice versa) and then flushed in sewer system after adding large quantity of water.

    It is to note that hospital liquid waste should never be discharged into natural water.

20. **What is lagooning?**
    Collection of water in large ponds which are with sedimentation devices. It provides settlement and further biological improvement through storage in large man-made ponds.

21. **What is effluent treatment plant (ETP)?**
    This is stepwise process of treating the effluent produced in the hospital.

22. **What are the advantages of ETP?**
    - Effluent water can be used for irrigation, sanitary purposes, etc.
    - Multidrug resistant bacterial are completely inactivated
    - Physiochemical parameters of effluent water remain within the acceptable limit
    - Sludge which is a byproduct can be used as manure
    - ETP is cost effective and environment friendly.

23. **What are the components of ETP and their function?**
    - Bar screen—removal of course suspended particles
    - Oil and grease trap—removal of oil and grease
    - Collection and equalization tank—collection and equalization of raw effluent

- Aeration tank—mixing of effluent with excess of air to remove the organic matter
- Clarifier tank—separates suspended biological material from effluent and returned to aeration tank and excess to sludge tank
- Filter feed tank—treated effluent is stored before passing to pressure and filter
- Pressure sand filter—removes fine suspended particles from treated effluent
- Chlorination tank—continuous chlorination of treated effluent
- Clean treated water tank—collection of clean treated water before final use
- Sludge tank—filling of sludge for drying and later use as manure.

24. **What should be the process for disposal for the waste generated during mass immunization program at outreach area or subcenters ?**

The given flowchart should be followed for proper waste management:

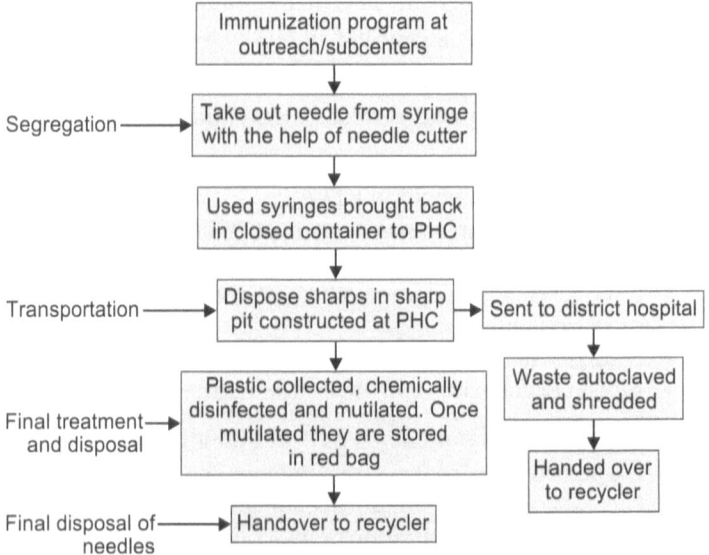

25. **What are the challenges of immunization waste in India?**
    The challenges in India to manage immunization waste are:
    - Remote locations of immunization program where sparse facilities are available
    - Though the waste quantity will be less but it will be scattered because of remotely located places
    - Scarcity of availability of needle cutter and mutilators
    - Transportation of waste from remote areas to primary health center (PHC) and other higher centers
    - Training of the available staff
    - Nonavailability of staff who have been trained because of various trivial reasons
    - Lack of motivation and low morale of the staff.

26. **What are the types of biomedical waste generated during Revised National Tuberculosis Control Program (RNTCP)?**
    The variety of waste generated during RNTCP are:
    - Human biological waste (sputum)
    - Use cotton swabs/guage pads
    - Laboratory waste
    - Drung packing material (general packing/blister packing)
    - Plastic waste
    - General waste (liquid waste, paper waste, broomsticks, discarded cloth pieces, discarded articles)
    - Constuction waste (waste generated from civil work activities).

27. **What are the challenges in RNTCP regarding biomedical waste?**
    Following are the challenges:
    - Safe disposal of sharps
    - Safe destruction of syringes with needles
    - Prevention of burning of plastic materials especially those which are preburning treated with chlorine producing chemicals
    - Ensuring that all concerned staff adopt to standard precautions in handling specimen and samples so as to avoid spillage
    - Ensuring deep and secured burial of used sputum cups and specimen slides.

Management of Specialized Waste

28. How the used slides in laboratory are managed?

The used slide are not broken into pieces before disposal but they are first disinfected by immersing in 5% phenol or 40% phenolic compound which is diluted to 5%. The duration for which they remain immersed is minimum 30 minutes. Later they are disoposed off with other hospital waste sharp in pit designated for sharps. The used chemical solution will be drained away in the hospital drainage system.

29. What are the steps involved in disposal of sputum cups and wooden sticks?

The essential steps are:

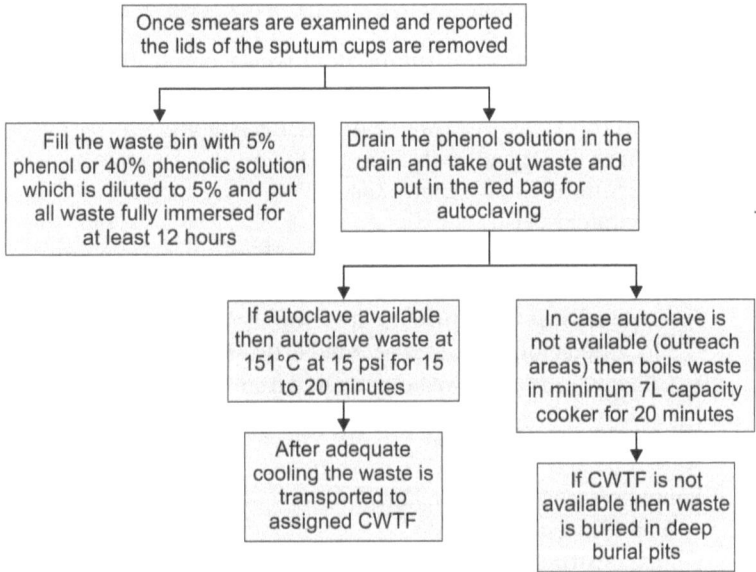

30. How the lead shields/lead foils are managed?

Lead is a heavy metal and lead foils and shields are present in the pure form. Lead is potentially hazardous to neurological system development and functioning. It can leach from landfills into the environment hence managed as hazardous material or lead shields and foils can be sent to metal recovery system.

Chapter 15

Cytotoxic Waste Management

1. **What is cytotoxic waste?**
   Cytotoxic waste is the byproduct of cytotoxic drug therapy which is administered to patients.

2. **What all is included in cytotoxic waste?**
   It includes all drug administrative equipment like needles, syringes, dripsets, left over cytotoxic medicine, etc. Besides this all gowns and body fluids/waste from patients undergoing such treatment also included in this category of waste.

3. **What are cytotoxic agents and what are their adverse effects on the body?**
   Cytotoxic agents are the substances used in the treatment of malignant and other diseases. They are designed to destroy rapidly growing cancerous cells in the body. They can develop mutagenic, carcinogenic and/or teratogenic effects on the body either in treatment doses or animal and bacterial assays.

4. **What are the types of effects of cytotoxic agents?**
   Cytotoxics agents can cause short-term to long-term effects on the human body ranging from irritation or allergic reactions to mutagenic, carcinogenic, and teratogenic effects.

5. **How one can get exposed to cytotoxic agents?**
   The exposure to cytotoxic agents may occur through skin contact, skin absorption, inhalation of aerosols, ingestion and needle stick injuries. At workplace personal contamination may result from the following activities. Agent preparation, agent administration, handling patient waste, transport and waste disposal or spills.

Cytotoxic Waste Management

6. **What action to be taken in the event of personal contamination with cytotoxic agent?**

   Immediately remove gloves or gown and any other contaminated clothing and dispose off in purple cytotoxic waste container. In case of clothing which are not overtly contaminated then they should undergo packaging and laundering before next use.

7. **What is to be done when there is direct eye, skin or other body contact with these agents?**

   Procedure need to be followed:
   - **Skin exposure**
     - Remove contaminated clothing immediately
     - Wash the affected skin thoroughly with plenty of running water.
   - **Eye exposure**
     - Immediately wash the eye with clean water by continuous irrigation for a period of 15 minutes.
   - **Needle stick injuries**
     - Wash thoroughly the pricked area as explained the process for skin exposure
     - If the needle stick injury results in the injection of agents, it may be necessary to refer to hospital guidelines for such incidences
     - Do not administer antiseptic or anesthetic drops or ointments on/in the pricked area.

8. **How the incidence is reported?**

   The process of incidence reporting is like:
   - In case of staff gets affected:
     - Immediately intimate superior staff
     - Visit emergency area
     - Complete incidence reporting.
   - In case patient gets affected:
     - Intimate superiors of the medical team
     - Duly fill up the incidence form and submit to administrative office.

9. **How many types of spills are there for cytotoxic agent spill?**

   There can be two types of spills less than 50 mL (minor) and more than 50 mL spill (major). This distinction is important because the methodology of management differ for these two types of spills.

Cytotoxic Waste Management

10. **When these spills can occur?**
    Spill can occur at the time of chemotherapy drug administration, during patient care and/or during patient or agent transport from one place to another.

11. **How the cytotoxic spill is managed?**
    The steps are as follow:
    - Isolate the area with tape and put sinage
    - Call hazardous materials (HAZMAT) team
    - Wear personal protective equipment (PPE) as required
    - Cover spill with tissue paper and pour detergent solution over it
    - Collect the whole soaked tissue papers and put it in yellow bag
    - Wash the area thoroughly with plenty of water
    - Dry the area, remove PPE and put them in yellow bag
    - Duly fill incidence form and submit to the concerned department.

12. **What should be done with excess cytotoxic agent?**
    Excess cytotoxic agent may occur in two situations:
    1. Agent or medication which has not been used and this portion must be returned back to pharmacy with due documentation.
    2. Left over part of administered (unused portion of used medication) medicine and this portion must be disposed off in yellow bag.

13. **How linen can get contaminated from cytotoxic agent?**
    Linen can get contaminated with nonactivated agent or activated metabolite of the inactive agent.

14. **What are cytotoxic drugs?**
    These are the therapeutic agents which are intended for, but not limited to the treatment of cancer. These drugs are highly toxic to cell due to their action on cell reproduction. They are used in noncancerous conditions as well, e.g. drug methotrexate is used in management of rheumatoid arthritis. Cytotoxic agents are also used in autoimmune disorders and multiple sclerosis.

15. **Which are the activities when the staff can get exposure to cytotoxic drugs?**
    - Drug admixing
    - Drug administration

- Transport of active drug from one place to another
- Handling patient waste
- Handling unused drug for disposal
- Drug spills (major or minor)

16. **Who all can get affected by these cytotoxic drugs?**
    The category of affected people are:
    - Pharmacists
    - Clinicians
    - Nurses
    - Laboratory staff
    - Housekeeping staff
    - Biomedical waste handling staff.

17. **What are the effects of cytotoxic drug on body?**
    The abnormal effects of these drugs on body are:
    - Mutagenic activity leading to abnormal formation of cells
    - Congenital malformation or fetal loss if pregnant woman get exposed to these drugs
    - Hair loss, loss of taste
    - Abdominal pain and vomiting
    - Contact dermatitis, allergic reaction
    - Local toxic effects
    - Liver damage.

18. **What is the minimum exposure of cytotoxic drug needed to produce effects?**
    There is no set dose limit of exposure to produce adverse effects as even the single exposure may cause drastic effects.

19. **At what time the exposure risk is maximum?**
    The maximum risk of exposure is at the time of chemotherapy admixing.

20. **How the risks of exposure to healthcare workers be reduced?**
    Following measure will help to reduce the risk from exposure:
    - Laid down protocols for personal safety
    - Strict implementation of safety protocols
    - Effective workplace planning and designing
    - Use of safety cabinet for drug admixing
    - Compliance to PPE while handling cytotoxic drugs
    - Integrated health monitoring program.

21. **What is the objective of integrated health monitoring program?**
    The objectives is to provide safety to the healthcare worker from adverse effects of cytotoxic drugs.

22. **How this objective can be achieved?**
    The objective can be achieved by:
    - Pre-employment assessement and counseling to prospective employees
    - Orientation and education about cytotoxic drugs.

23. **How the risk from cytotoxic waste can be reduced?**
    It can be reduced by implementing following strategies:
    - Hazard identification
    - Cytotoxic waste assessment
    - Personal management
    - Documentation of activities related to interaction with cytotoxic material
    - Regular training to concerned staff
    - Periodic review of the activities.

24. **When the training related to safety from cytotoxic material be given?**
    It should be given at the time of:
    - Employee induction program
    - When new equipment is placed or there is change in procedures
    - Prior to commencement of duties leading to handling of cytotoxic materials.

25. **Who need training in cytotoxic material handling?**
    They are:
    - Nursing staff
    - Pharmacy staff
    - Cytotoxic waste handlers and transporters
    - Laboratory staff members
    - Waste handlers.

26. **What topics in training should cover?**
    The information related to cytotoxic drugs and related waste should cover:
    - Occupational hazards of cytotoxic exposures
    - Health risk related to waste
    - Control measures

- Equipment maintenance
- Access to first aid/emergency services
- Correct and appropriate selection of PPE
- Measures to be taken in case of accidental exposures
- Storage, transport, treatment and disposal of cytoxic waste.

26. **How the training program is evaluated?**
    The training program is evaluated though various methodologies which are:
    - Assessment of improvement in the work performance
    - Monitoring of work practices
    - Analysis of the incidences.

27. **Which is the best way to control the drug exposures?**
    Use of ready to use drug form, e.g. prefilled syringes.

28. **What is the standard operating procedure (SOP) for preparation of cytotoxic drug in the healthcare setting?**
    The SOP should mention that:
    - The glass ampoules must be broken with ampoule breaker
    - Use dedicated equipment to prepare drug
    - Use PPE while preparing drug
    - Use diluted drug whenever possible
    - Use sharp waste container to avoid exposures.

29. **When one can get exposed to cytotoxic waste?**
    Following are the situations when one can get exposed to the waste:
    - Handling blood and body fluids
    - Handling vomitus, urine, excreta and fluid drained from the body cavities
    - Handling bedpans, urinary catheter bags, colostomy/urostomy bags and urinals
    - Handling patient's linen or clothings contaminated with cytotoxic drug or waste
    - While cleaning the spills.

30. **What should contained in the cytotoxic waste management policy?**
    The organization should place policy regarding cytotoxic waste management and ensue compliance to the same. Designate the staff who will be responsible to ensure the waste disposal in most efficient way from segration to the final disposal (from cradle to grave). Waste management audit to be carried out regularly.

31. **How the bags for cytotoxic waste collection is identified?**
    The bag is of purple color with symbol of cell in the late phase of cell division called telophase. The container is identified by the words "cytotoxic waste".

32. **How the spill of the cytotoxic powder is managed?**
    The powder should be covered with tissue paper, taking care that tissue paper does not cause dust production in 3-4 layers and carefully wet the paper so that powder dissolves. Now collect the abosorbed material carefully and discard into the yellow bags.

33. **What is to be done in case the cytotoxic drug goes into eyes?**
    Immediately wash the affected eye with plenty of clean water with the help of continuous irrigation for atleast 15 minutes. Care is taken not to put any drops or ointment into affected eye. Prepare incidence report and submit to the concerned authority of the hospital.

34. **How the cytotoxic waste be collected at the point of generation?**
    Staff should keep all contaminated syringes, IV lines, bottles at one place. Care should be taken not to disconnect line from the bag. Put them all in the yellow bag carefully so that there is no exposure or spillage.

35. **What is the most hazardous duration post drug administration?**
    After drug administration next 48 hours are most hazardous period for drug excretion though many drug keep on getting excreted up to 7 days.

36. **What precaution staff should take during this period?**
    Staff should take following precautions:
    - Follow universal precautions
    - Patient should be advised to flush the toilet with the lid down
    - Open articles should be sanitized as soon as possible
    - If there is time for doing the sanitization for these article then they should be covered with absorbent paper and everyone should know about it.
    - Reusable equipments should be washed immediately with soap and warm water and must not left to be cleaned by another staff.

37. **How reduction in cytotoxic waste can be achieved?**
    It can be achieved through three methodologies:
    - Product substitution (in place of toxic product use non toxic or less toxic product)
    - Product modification
    - Procedural change.

38. **Why urine of patient post drug be disposed carefully?**
Because the urine may contain high concentration of active drug or hazardous metabolites. Care should be taken in case patient has receive intravesical chemotherapy or one who have received high doses of drug which primarily get excreted in the urine as unchanged or as active metabolite. It is advisable for concerned staff to adhere to universal precautions.

39. **How to manage linen which are contaminated with cytotoxic waste?**
The linen contaminated with patient's blood, body fluid, excreta who have received drug in last 48 hours or spilled drugs are hazardous and must be handled carefully. Before they are put with other linen for washing they must be prewashed with soap and plenty of water.

40. **What should be the contents of incidence form in case of cytotoxic drug exposure?**
The main contents are:
- Date and time of incident
- Location of the incident
- Name of the drug
- Form of the drug (liquid, powder, etc.)
- Concentration of the drug (pure or diluted)
- Approximate quantity of spill
- Name of the staff members exposed
- Area of the body exposure
- Description of corrective and preventive action (CAPA)

41. **What does this sign signify?**
This sign signifies the cytotoxic waste.

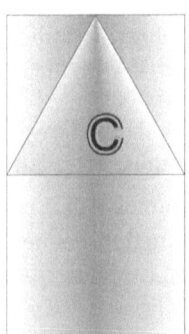

Chapter 16

Disinfectants in Hospital

1. **What is the difference between disinfections, sterilization, disinfectants, antiseptics, sanitizers, and decontamination?**

   Disinfections: It is the process of killing microorganisms, but not usually spores, for prevention or control of infectious disease

   Sterilization: It is the process of destruction of all the microorganisms including spores from materials and making them bacteria free

   Disinfectants: These are the germicidal agents capable of destroying micro-organisms but not necessarily their spores. Due to their toxic nature, they are used only for disinfections of inanimate objects

   Antiseptics: When disinfectants are suitably diluted so as to suitable for human requirements they are called antiseptics. Due to nontoxic nature they are recommended for superficial application of human tissue

   Senitizers: These are the substances which reduce the number of microorganisms to a safe level

   Decontamination: It is the process removal of disease producing microorganisms to leave an item safe for further handling.

2. **What are the types of disinfections?**
   - *Concurrent disinfection*: When the disinfection is carried out in the presence of infectious patients. For example, linen clothes, dressing material, gloves, instruments, etc.
   - *Terminal disinfections*: When disinfection is carried out after the discharge or death of the patients. For example, bedding, linen soiled cloths, etc.

3. **What is the difference between disinfectant and sanitizer?**
The disinfectant at a specified dilution has higher pathological microbacterial killing capability than sanitizer.

4. **What are the principle guidelines for disinfectants?**
   - Use of particulars type of disinfectant for particular purpose
   - Dilution of disinfectant
   - Contact time of particular disinfectant
   - Safety aspects for disinfectant
   - Frequency of use of disinfectant.

5. **What are the properties of disinfectant?**
   - Inexpensive and noncorrosive
   - Offers complete sterilization
   - Has wide spectrum of activities
   - It is nontoxic.

6. **What factors affect the potency of a disinfectant?**
   - Dilution reduces the potency of a disinfectant
   - Presence of organic materials
   - Chemical nature of disinfectants
   - Degree of contamination
   - Contact time and temperature
   - pH and interaction with other compounds.

7. **What is phenol coefficient?**
This is the relative effectiveness of a disinfectant when compared to that of phenol. To measure the phenol coefficient *S. typhi* or *S. aureus* microbes are used. If the disinfectant is more effective than phenol then the coefficient is >1 and those disinfectant which are less effective have coefficient <1.

8. **What are noncritical, semi-critical and critical items (instrument/devices) used in patient care?**
Noncritical items: These are the items which come in contact with intact skin but not mucous membrane or do not directly contact the patients.
   The disinfections done by cleaning and/or low level disinfection.
Semi-critical item: These are the items which come in contact with nonintact skin or mucous membrane but non-necessarily penetrate them.

The disinfection done by meticulous cleaning followed by high level disinfections.

Critical items: These are instruments or devices which enter sterile tissues including the vascular system.

The disinfections involve meticulous cleaning followed by sterilization because of high-risk of infection.

9. **What are the levels of disinfections?**
   - Low level disinfection
   - Intermediate level disinfection
   - High level disinfection.

10. **What is the criteria for this classification?**
    The level of disinfections done by any disinfectants is based on the basis of cidal (killing) activity for microorganism.

11. **Describe in brief low, intermediate and high level disinfectants.**
    Low level disinfectants: These disinfectants kill most vegetative bacteria and some fungi and evolved (lipid) virus like HBV, HCV, HIV but do not kill spores and mycobacteria. These disinfectants are used to clean environmental surfaces.

    Intermediate level disinfectants: These disinfectants kill vegetative bacteria and most of virus and fungi but not resistant bacterial spores.

    High level disinfectants: Kill vegetative bacteria, fungi and viruses but not necessarily spores.

12. **Which alcohols are used as disinfectants and what are disadvantages?**
    - Ethanol (Ethyl alcohol)
    - Isopropyl alcohol

    Disadvantages:
    - Fire hazards
    - Limited residual activity due to evaporation
    - Brief contact time
    - Limited activity in the presence of organic material.

13. **Why alcohols are more effective when combined with purified water?**
    Because higher water content allows greater diffusion through cell membrane and that is why 70% alcohol is more effective than 90% alcohol.

14. **What is the mechanism action of oxidizing agents?**
    Oxidizing agent oxidises the cell membrane of microorganisms thus causing loss of structure leading to lyses of cells.

15. **Give examples of oxidizing agents.**
    - Sodium hypochlorite
    - Hydrogen paroxide
    - Chloramine
    - Iodine
    - Peracetic acid.

16. **Give examples of low level, intermediate level and high level disinfectants.**
    Low level disinfectants:
    - Phenol
    - Quaternary amorous compounds.

    Intermediate level disinfectants:
    - Alcohols
    - Hypochlorite
    - Iodophores.

    High level disinfactants:
    - Hydrogen peroxide
    - Formaldehyde
    - Glutoraldehyde
    - Peracetic acid.

17. **What are the advantages and disadvantages of sodium hypochlorite?**
    Advantages:
    - Rapid action
    - Broad range of activity
    - Low cost
    - Unaffected by water hardness
    - Low incidence of serious toxicity.

    Disadvantages:
    - Presence of organic matters makes than ineffective
    - Chemical instability because chlorine is lost rapidly
    - Corrosive
    - Imitating at high concentration.

18. **What are iodophores?**
    Iodophore is a combination of carrier and iodine and this carrier allows continuous release of iodine in small amounts. The cidal

action of iodophores is due to disruption of protein and nucleic acid structure and their synthesis. The iodophores have two main demerits:
1. Plastic and rubber items get discolored or stained
2. Metallic items get corroded when disinfected for prolonged period.

19. **What are quaternary ammonium compounds?**
These compounds are low level disinfectants and contain NH_4^+ and as they contain strong positive charge they make easy contact with negatively charged surface and this makes them very good cleaning agents. These compounds are not effective against non-enveloped virus, fungi and spores.
Merits:
- Low toxicity
- Good cleaning agents.

Demerits:
- Ineffective in presence of hard water
- Irritating on prolonged contact
- Less microbicidal in presence of organic matters.

20. **Give examples of concentration of disinfectant used.**

Lysol	2%
Sodium hypochlorite	1%
Glutaraldehyde	2%
Isopropyl alcohol	70%
Hydrogen peroxide	3%

21. **What is the common name of sodium hypochlorite?**
Household bleach (4-6% sodium hypochlorite).

22. **What steps should be taken to prevent the environmental pollution from disinfectants?**
   - Select the right product
   - Frequency of disinfection to be kept minimum
   - Use of controlled product mix as per the direction of manufactures (usual dilution is 1 part concentrated disinfectant in 125-500 parts of water)
   - Use correct method of using disinfectant so as to use it effectively at lower concentration and in less quantity.

23. **What are the advantages of ortho-phthalaldehyde (OPA) over glutaraldehyde?**
    OPA has following advantages:
    - Excellent stability over wide range from pH 3 to pH 9
    - Not irritant to mucous membrane of eyes and nasal cavity
    - Does not require exposure monitoring
    - Needs no activation.

24. **What is ortho-phthaladehyde (OPA)?**
    It is a highly potent disinfectant used for thermolabile and thermostable instruments.

25. **How it is used?**
    It is ready to use solution and does not need any activation or dilution.

26. **For which instruments this can be used?**
    It can be used for instruments like flexible and rigid endoscopes, laproscopes, anesthesia and dental equipments.

27. **What is the prerequisite for use of OPA?**
    The instruments needs to be thoroughly cleaned, rinsed and almost dried.

28. **What is after using OPA for instruments?**
    The instruments are thoroughly cleaned before use.

29. **What are the microbiological properties of OPA?**
    It is a rapidly acting microbicidal agent. It's activity is against viruses (envelope and nonenvelope), fungi and vegetative organisms.

30. **What precautions should one take while using OPA?**
    It is harmful by inhalation, ingestion and for skin contacts. The place where it is being used should be well ventilated, the user should used protective glasses and gloves, etc.

31. **What is the duration of OPA high level disinfection?**
    12 minutes of duration for the instrument should remain immersed.

32. **For how many days it can be reused?**
    For maximum 14 days then it is discarded. The unused solution can be kept for 75 days in tightly lid container.

33. **How chlorhexidine can be used in the hospitals?**
    It can be used for hand antisepsis and surgical hand antisepsis. The duration of time for former is 30 seconds while for latter it is 1.5–3 minutes. For skin antisepsis before surgical procedure allow it to dry for up to 30 seconds.

34. **What are microbiological properties of chlorhexidine?**
    It is active against Gram positive as well as Gram negative bacteria.

35. **What concentration of hydrogen peroxide be used for surface disinfectant and fogging purpose?**
    For surface disinfection it is used in 10% concentration while for fogging purpose required concentration is 20%.

36. **Where all the surface and environmental disinfectant are used?**
    The areas where it is used are operation theater (OT), intensive care units (ICUs), wards, consulting rooms, and dressing rooms, etc.

37. **What is the contact period for surface disinfection?**
    For critical care area it is 1 hour while for other areas is 30 minutes.

38. **What concentration is used for critical and noncritical area?**
    For critical areas 2% solution (dissolve 200 mL solution in 10 liters of water) and for noncritical area the concentration is 0.5% (50 mL solution in 10 liters of water).

39. **What are the most common chemical used in hospitals?**
    These are:
    - Gluteraldehyde
    - Phenolics
    - Xylene (dimethylebenzene, xylol)
    - Mercury
    - Methyl methacrylate.

40. **What is the criteria for glutaraldehyde waste disposal?**
    Glutaraldehyde is mainly disposed in sewer provided it is diluted below 0.1% concentration and the total quantity to be disposed off limited to 50 L of 2% of glutaraldehyde per day.

41. **How HIV can be deactivated?**
    HIV can be deactivated by the use of various chemicals.

Chemicals	Percentage of chemicals	Remarks
Glutaraldehyde	2%	Available as CIDEX
Formaldehyde	5%	Prepared by dissolving 50 g in 1 L
Hydrogen peroxide	3%	—
Ethanol	70%	Prepared by dissolving 700 g in 1 L
Household bleach	1%	Available as 3-5% readymade solution. Prepared by dissolving 2.5 volumes of tap water to ready made solution to get 1% solution
Isopropyl alcohol	35%	—
Dysol	0.5%	—
Tween 20	2.5%	—

42. **How much time does it take to deactivate HIV by boiling water?**
    HIV is deactivated by boiling water in seconds.

43. **How much time a disinfectant takes to act?**
    Minimum 10 min or more. On the surface apply disinfactant and leave it for 10 min or more.

44. **What are the steps for disinfection?**
    There are four steps for the process of disinfection:
    Step 1: Precleaning is the most important step and in this the surface is cleaned water and soap. The precleaning is required because presence of dust on surface may harbor microbs.
    Step 2: Application of disinfectant on surface.
    Step 3: Wipe off the disinfectant because disinfectant may leave sticky stains which may further deposit microbs.
    Step 4: Cleaning of surface with water and drying of with tissue paper.

45. **What is the difference between bleach and non bleach disinfectant?**
    Non bleach disinfectants only sanitize the applied surface and good for clothes and delicate surfaces. On the other hand bleach disinfectants are commonly used for hard surfaces of bathrooms and kitchen. They should bot be used for delicate

surface like skin. While using bleach disinfectants user should wear the mask, gloves and keep open the windows for exit of harmful vapours.

46. **What precautions should be used while using bleach disinfectants?**

    Any item which has come in contact with should either be discarded or washed with plenty of water and sundried.

47. **What is difference between cleaning, sanitization and disinfection?**

    Cleaning: It is the process of removing visible debris, dust and dirt from the surface. At the same time it bears the risk of cross contamination through mopping solution and cleaning tools.

    Sanitization: It is the process of reducing occurrence and growth of bacteria, viruses and fungi on the surface. It reduces number of bacterial presence by 99.9 percent.

    Disinfection: It is the process which will kill the microbes.

    Suppose there are one million organisms on surface then sanitiser will reduce number of oragnisms down to 1000 but nothing about fungus and virus but disinfectant will kill 100 percent organisms.

48. **When the hand sanitizer is useful?**

    It is more useful during traveling, camping, in shcools, colleges, and public transportation.

49. **How many types of hand sanitizers are available?**

    Two types of hand sanitizers are available—one is alcohol based and another is alcohol free sanitizers.

50. **What is the usual percentage of alcohol in alcohol based hand sanitizer?**

    The percentage of alcohol is 60-65% and it kills 99.9% microbacteria. Higher the percentage of alcohol, higher will have germicidal action.

51. **Through which phenomenon alcohol works?**

    Alcohol works on phenomenon of friction. The alcohol has low boiling point. So when hands are rubbed the warmth, which is generated due to friction of palms or fingers, evaporates alcohol which takes germs particles with them.

52. Why alcohol free sanitizers are not preferred?

Because alcohol free hand sanitizers are less effective as germicidal though they don't cause skin dryness like alcohol based saniziters.

53. What is the main content of alcohol free hand sanitizers?

These sanitizers contain quaternary ammonium compounds called benzalkonium chloride.

Chapter 17

Biomedical Waste Management in COVID-19

1. **What name WHO announced for corona virus?**
   SARS Corona Virus -2.

2. **Why it called corona?**
   The name corona has been derived from the outer fringe, or "corona" of embedded envelope protein. It looks like a crown hence named.

3. **What is the name of disease caused by corona virus?**
   COVID-19.

4. **What is COVID?**
   Corona virus disease.

5. **what was previous name of COVID19**
   2019 Novel Corona Virus.

6. **Why there are different name of virus and disease?**
   Virus name is based on genetic structure to facilitate diagnostic test, vaccines and medicines. Diseases are named to enable workers on disease prevention, transmissibility, severity and treatment.

7. **How the humans get infected with this virus?**
   Primary way of infection is from person to person transmission. The close contact of person may be from hug, handshake or being in crowed space like bus, tram, local train or congregation etc.

8. **How secretions spread infection?**
   The infected individual easily spread droplets which coughing or sneezing which can be taken up by other person who is in close proximity.

The droplets are heavy so easily and quickly fall on ground and based on the type of surface they fall they remain there before being touched by hand which then carries them to other parts of the body like nose, mouth, eye or to another individual by handshake, etc.

9. **How cough contributes in spread of infection?**
   A single cough can produce up to 3,000 droplets. These particles can land on other people, clothing and surfaces around them, but some of the smaller particles can remain in the air.

10. **How long virus survives on the hard surface?**
    As per CDC the survival of virus on cardboard is up to 24 hours and up to 2-3 days on plastic and stainless-steel surfaces.

11. **Which is the best way to remove virus form hand?**
    Frequent hand washing with soap and water. This is simple and effective method because it is extremely destructive to virus. A drop of soap diluted in water is sufficient to rupture and kill virus. However after washing hands should be dried with disposable tissue paper.

12. **Why soap is very disruptive to virus?**
    The soap is disruptive because of its molecule has hybrid structure. The soap molecule is pin shaped where head is hydrophilic (affinity for water) hence bonds with water and hydrophobic trail (avoid water) hence bonds with oil and fats.

13. **What is the mechanism of action of soap?**
    The soap molecules, when get suspended in water, float as independent unit and these units interact with other molecules in the solution and assemble into tiny bubbles which are called micelles. In the micelles the head points outwards and tail point inwards. When hands are rinsed the trapped virus, bacteria and dirt is washed away.

14. **What are the viruses having lipid membrane as their envelop?**
    Corona, HIV, Hepatitis B and C, herpes, Ebola, Zica and Dengue.

15. **How sanitizers work?**
    Sanitizers contain about 60% alcohol and act by destabilizing lipid membrane present in virus and bacteria. Also the alcohol has the ability to unfold and inactivate their proteins and this process is known as denaturation.

16. **What is the limitations with sanitizers?**
    Sanitizers can not easily remove microorganisms from skin. Also some viruses don't depend on lipid membranes but have shields of proteins and sugars.

17. **Why does WHO recommend hand rub?**
    WHO recommends hand rub because of following reasons:
    - Broad spectrum of antimicrobial activity
    - Suitable for remote and resource scarcity locations
    - Because of easy availability and faction compliance to hand hygiene is increased
    - Economic because of cost reduction
    - If many patients are to be touched in short time.

18. **What is the correct way to use hand rub?**
    WHO has given the guidelines on using hand rub and these can be Mnemonic as TRAPS.
    T—Tips of fingers
    R—rub hand as palm to palm and dorsum of hand to palm
    A—adequate amount sanitizer
    P—proper time spent sanitizing (15–30 sec)
    S—spray in between the fingers

19. **What are the advantages of hand wash over use of sanitizers?**
    Following are points in favor of hand wash:
    - It cleans away the residue
    - Does not over dry the skin
    - There is no allergic reaction to which is common due to alcohol.

20. **How to get rid of dryness of hand after frequent cleaning?**
    Use of good quality moistures with take care of dryness of hands.

21. **What are the areas of biomedical waste generation during Corona Epidemic?**
    The biomedical waste will be generated during diagnosis and treatment of COVID-19 suspected and confirmed cases in:
    - Isolation wards
    - Quarantine centers
    - Sample collection room
    - Camps
    - Urban local bodies (ULBs)
    - Laboratories
    - Common treatment facility (CTF).

22. **Who should be reported about opening of COVID-19 ward?**
    State pollution control board should be reported regarding opening of COVID-19 ward.

23. **What is the mechanism for biomedical waste management (BMWM) in isolation ward?**
    Following steps are important:
    - Keep color codes bins as per BMWM Rules 2016
    - Use double layered yellow colored bags to ensure no leaks and adequate strength of collection bags
    - Bags should be labeled "COVID-19 waste" and stored separately before handing over to common biomedical treatment facility (CBWTF). This would help the facility to identify waste for priority treatment and immediate disposal
    - Maintain separate record of "COVID19 waste"
    - Dedicated separate trolleys to be used for transportation and storage of waste
    - The trolley's outer and inner surfaces must be cleaned with 1% sodium hypochlorite solution.

24. **What is the mechanism for BMWM in quarantine camps/home care?**
    Following steps are important:
    - Biomedical waste be collected in double layered yellow colored bag
    - Intimate CBWTF for collection of waste directly form source
    - In **home care** waste is collected in yellow bag and directly handed over to authorized waste collector engaged by local bodies. This can be done as home to home collection or identified central collection point.

25. **What is the mechanism for BMWM in CBWTF?**
    Following steps are important:
    - Report to state pollution control board (SPCB)/pollution control committee (PCCs) about receiving COVID-19 waste from various sources
    - Regular thorough sanitization of workers
    - All workers to be provided with PPE (3 layer mask, eye shield, nitril gloves, gumboots, splash proof gowns)
    - Use dedicated vehicle for transportation of COVID19 waste
    - Vehicle should be sanitized with 1% sodium hypochlorite or other appropriate chemical disinfectant after every collection trip

- COVID-19 waste should be disposed of immediately
- Facility should inform SPCBs if it needs to operate for extra hours due to waste load
- Facility should maintain COVID-19 waste record for collection, treatement and disposal.
- If any employee showing features of illness then that staff should immediately be isolated and be sent on leave till free from illness.

26. **What are the duties of SPCBs and PCCs?**

    The duties of SPCBs and PCCs are as below:
    - Should maintain the records of COVID-19 treatment wards, quarantine centers and home cares
    - Ensure proper collection and disposal of waste as per guidelines
    - Monitor working of CBWTF
    - Permit CBWTF to collect waste from quarantine camps which otherwise don't qualify as healthcare facility.

27. **What are the steps of cleaning of hands with hand rub?**

    The process of hand hygiene with hand rub can be done in 7 steps as shown in photograph below:

7 steps of handwashing with hand sanitizer

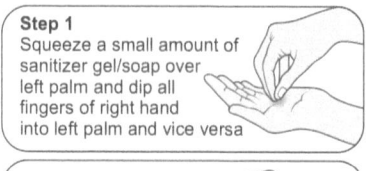

Step 1
Squeeze a small amount of sanitizer gel/soap over left palm and dip all fingers of right hand into left palm and vice versa

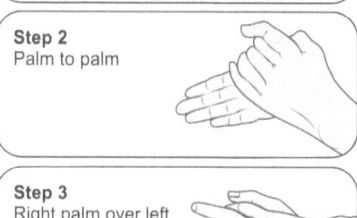

Step 2
Palm to palm

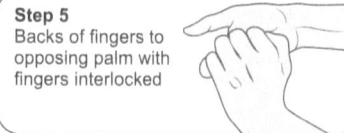

Step 5
Backs of fingers to opposing palm with fingers interlocked

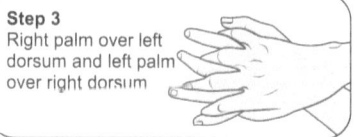

Step 3
Right palm over left dorsum and left palm over right dorsum

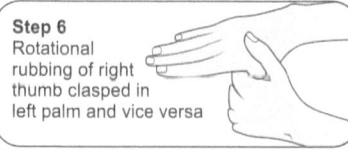

Step 6
Rotational rubbing of right thumb clasped in left palm and vice versa

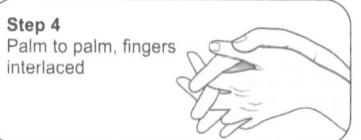

Step 4
Palm to palm, fingers interlaced

Step 7
Rotational rubbing of right wrist and vice vers.
Rinse and dry thoroughly

Key Concepts

Acceptable risk: It is the risk with minimal detrimental effects. This can also be defined as the risk in which benefits outweigh the potential hazards.

Accreditation: A process of external review of the quality of the healthcare being provided by health care organization (HCO). This process generally carried by nonprofit nongovernment organization (NGO). Accreditation mean the organization meet an applicable set of standards.

Act: A statute or law adopted (enacted) by a national or state legislative or other governing body. Act is distinguished from resolutions where latter is used to express legislative opinion or to regulate affairs of the governing body itself, and from ordinance or by laws of municipal corporation and rules and regulations of administrations.

Acute: Occurance over a short time say within few minutes or hours. An acute exposure can lead to short-term but sometimes long-term health effects.

Acute toxicity: Where a toxic effect occurs immediately or shortly after a single exposure.

Aeration: Method which helps in removal of ethylene oxide (EtO) from the items sterilized by EtO. This is achieved by circulation of warm air in enclosed cabinet specifically designed by this purpose.

Agent: An entity which may be chemical, biological, radiological which may cause effects in an organism exposed to these.

Air pollution: Presence of solid, liquid or gaseous substance in the atmosphere in such a concentration that it may be injurious to human beings and/or other living creatures or plants or property or environment.

Alcohol based formulation: An alcohol containing preparation (in the form of gel, foam or liquid) designed to be applied on hands for hand antisepsis in hygienic way.

Key Concepts

Antibiogram: The result of laboratory testing for the sensitivity of an isolated bacterial strain to different sets of antibiotics arranged in culture media.

Antineoplastic: Anti-cancer.

Antiseptic: A chemical agent used on the skin and mucous membrane so as to prevent growth and development, remove or to kill micro-organisms without causing damage or irritation to the tissues. They are not used on surfaces or instruments like disinfectants.

Asepsis: It is the state when there is freedom from infection or infectious (pathogenic) material.

Aseptic: Sterile, free from germs.

Aseptic procedure: Any procedure which is performed using aseptic technique.

Aseptic technique: It is the technique which is used during patient care so as to prevent micro-organisms on surfaces, hands and equipments from being introduce to susceptible sites. These unlike sterilization are bedside methods.

Assessment: The process of determining the extent and nature of hazards and health problem within a particular jurisdiction.

Atomic Energy Regulatory Board (AERB): Constituted on 15 November 1983 by the President of India to carry out certain regulatory and safety functions in the fields of nuclear and radiation safety on a countrywide basis. The board is entrusted with the responsibility of laying down safety standards, and framing rules and regulations covering regulatory and safety functions envisaged under the section 27 of Atomic Energy Act, 1962. The mission of the AERB is to ensure the use of ionizing radiation and nuclear energy in India does not cause undue risk to the health of people and the environment.

Audit: It is a review which determines the extent to which a process or performance conforms to predetermined criteria or standards.

Australia antigen (synonym with hepatitis B antigen): Known as so because it was first detected in Australian aborigine. It is a biomarker indicating prevalence of infection with hepatitis B virus.

Autoclaving: The process of destruction of micro-organisms by steam under pressure.

Bactericidal: Chemical agents which are capable of killing of bacteria.

Bacteriostatic: Chemical agents which inhibit the growth of bacteria but do not necessarily kill them.

Benchmarking: Process of comparing ones performance results to the industry's best in similar process exists, e.g. VAP, SSI, ALOS, etc.

Bioburden: The population of viable infectious agents contaminating a medical device.
Biodegradable: Any substance which can be broken down by biological processes through the action of bacteria and other organisms present in the nature.
Biohazard: Hazardous to life.
Biological indicator: It is the device used to monitor the process of sterilization. There is standardized and viable population of bacterial spores known to be resistant to sterilization which under monitoring. These indicator are intended to demonstrate whether conditions for sterilization process were adequate to achieve desired sterilization.
Body fluids: Secretions—tears, milk, colostrums, wax, mucous secretions, saliva, sperms, etc; exudates and transudates—CSF, lymphatic, pleural fluid, ascetic fluid, pus, articular fluid; excretions—urine, vomit, lochia, muconium, feces; organic samples—placenta, organs, tissues, etc.
Bundle: A set of evidence based practices which when performed collectively and consistently have been demonstrated to improve outcome. These are used to improve the care process and patient outcome.
Cancer: A malignant tumor which can spread to other organs of the body, distinct from a benign tumor which cannot. (Although leukemia and some other malignant diseases are not solid tumors, they meet other criteria for cancer and can be, and often are, included under this definition.)
Carcinogen: An agent which is responsible for the formation of cancer.
Carcinogenic: Capable of causing cancer.
Carrier: The individual in whom presence of pathogenic micro-organisms does not cause any clinical symptoms of infections or without signs of any immune response.
Checklist: Written informational aid used to minimize failure in task completion by compensating for limits of human attention and memory. It also helps in maintaining the consistency and completeness in carrying out the particular tasks. Example—checklist for spill management, checklist for waste management, audit checklist for waste generation.
Chemical disinfection: It the process which eliminates almost all recognized pathogenic organisms but not necessarily all microbial forms on surface or objects.

Chemical indicator: It is like biological indicator, also a device used for sterilization monitoring purpose. There would be characteristic physical or chemical change to one or more physical conditions within sterilization chamber. They intend to detect sterilization failures from any reason. This indicator shows that the item undergone process of sterilization but does not necessarily prove that the item is sterile. There are six classes of indicators—class 1 process indicators; class 2 Bowie-Dick test indicator; class 3 single parameter indicator; class 4 multiparameter indicator; class 5 integrating indicator and class 6 emulating indicator.

Chemotherapy: The use of any chemical agents to treat or control disease. Most often used to describe treatment of malignant and other diseases with cytotoxic agent.

Chronic toxicity: Harmful effects of a chemical which occur after repeated or prolonged exposure. Chronic effects may also occur some time after exposure has ceased.

Cleaning: The process which physically removes adherent visible soil, protein substances, soil, debris and micro-organisms contamination from the hands, surfaces, crevices, serrations, lumen, joints of device, instruments and equipments by mechanical or manual process but not necessarily destroy micro-organisms thus making safe for handling and/or further decontamination. This can be done either with detergent and water or enzyme cleaner and water.

Clinical governance: Systemic approach for improving and sustaining the quality of patient care within health system. According to definition the healthcare organization is accountable for continuous improvement in quality of their services and maintaining high standards of clinical care by creating an environment in the organization where excellence in clinical care will flourish.

Contact time: It is the time a disinfectant remains in direct contact with surface or item. For surface disinfection it is the time period from application of disinfectant to surface till complete drying has occurred.

Contaminant: Any substance that enters a system where it is not normally found.

Contamination: Soiling of inanimate objects or living material with harmful, potential infection or unwanted matter. Also the present of blood or body fluids, that may be infectious, on an item or surface.

Controlling: One of the managerial functions that helps in checking errors and to take corrective action so as to reduce any deviation from set standards therefore the objective of the organization are achieved in desired manner. In older time the concept of control used to come once error has occurred so its recurrence is prevented but in modern time the concept is change in foreseeing action. It can be summarized as process of setting standard then measuring actual performance and taking corrective action as and when needed.

CRBSI: Catheter related bloodstream infection also known as catheter related sepsis. This is defined as presence of bacteremia originating from IV catheter. It is the most common cause of HAI. Due to strict aseptic precautions the rate of CRBSI is reducing though use of central venous catheter is increasing. Overall rate is around 3% but may be high to around 16%, the cause may be peripheral and/or central cannulation. It is responsible for prolonged ALOS and increased cost of treatment also mortality rate up to 25%.

Critical care areas: Designated areas in the healthcare facility that provide specialized postsurgical treatment to extremely ill patients. These area are ICU, NICU, CCU, burn care units, stroke units, etc. In these areas the critical requirements are constant patient monitoring, rest to patients and prompt response to emergency if arises.

Critical items: Medical devices or instruments which enter the sterile tissues of the body including vascular system. These items pose high risk of infection in case they are used contaminated with any micro-organisms. They are processed by initial meticulous cleaning followed by sterilization.

Critically important antibiotics: Antibiotics which are especially important in treating people who have severe infections caused by resistant bacteria.

Critical sites: These are the sites which are associated with high-risk of infection hence need to be protected against micro-organisms.

Cross contamination: Also known as cross infection. It is the transfer of micro-organisms from one surface, medium or person to another surface, medium or person and capable of spreading infection in both.

Cytogenetics: The study of the structure and functions of the cells of the body, with particular reference to the chromosomes.

Cytotoxic: Destructive to living cells. An agent or process that is toxic to cells.

Dangerous material book: Also called material safety datasheet (MSDS). This is compilation of detailed information about the dangerous substances being used in healthcare settings. This book intended to provide procedures for handling those substances in safe manner so as not to affect health adversely. The contents of the book differ from one organization to another depending on used of materials. The details about the product, handling precautions, adverse effects on health and spillage management are described in the book with specification.

Data collection: Systemic gathering of various types of data from different sources to be used for a particular purpose. This one of the step of statistical analysis. Data can be collected through questionnaire, interview, available documents, etc.

Decontamination: A process which removes or destroys contamination therefore prevents micro-organisms or other contaminants reaching a susceptible site in sufficient quantities to initiate infection or any other harmful response. Three processes of decontamination are commonly used: cleaning, disinfection, sterilization.

Disinfection: It is the process which is used to reduce number of viable micro-organisms but may not necessarily inactivate some bacterial agents like bacterial spores and viruses.

Droplet: Small particles (1-10 um) of micro-organisms containing respiratory secretions expelled in to the air by activities like coughing, sneezing and these are reduced to small dried particles by virtue of evaporation. Dry residue can remain air borne for long time and spread diseases by droplet infections.

Drug interaction: Situation in which one drug affects the activity of another drug when these two drugs are administered simultaneously. The interaction may be antagonistic when drug's effects is reduced (chloramphenicol + cephalosporin) or synergistic when drug's effect is increased (clavulanic acid + amoxycillin).

Drug resistance: Reduction in effectiveness of a drug in curing a disease or condition. The resistance develop for the drugs (antibiotic) targeting only specific bacterial protein and if that protein is changed because of mutation then it will interfere with its destruction by the antibiotic thus resulting in antibiotic resistance.

Endotoxin: Is a toxin lipopolysaccharide, formed by the breakdown of the cell wall of gram-negative bacteria. The endotoxin can be active even if the toxin releasing bacteria is killed.

Epidemic: A sudden increase in the incidence of cases of a particular disease, rapidly reaching a peak and then declining to low or undetectable levels. During epidemic the disease usually spread beyond the population in which the disease is normally endemic.

Epidemiology: Study of factors which influence the occurrence, frequency and distribution of a disease or infection in defined population.
Evaluation: Systemic determination of process significance, merits or worthiness using criteria those are governed by a predecided set of standards. It assists in identification of future change.
Excreta: Any waste matter eliminated from the body.
Exposure time: It is the time period, during the process of sterilization, for which items are exposed to the sterilant at the specified sterilization parameters. The parameter for example in autoclave is temperature.
Extravasation: Leakage of cytotoxic drug from the vein into the surrounding tissue.
Flash sterilization: Process used for steam sterilization of items for immediate use. The items in this process are kept in container unwrapped.
Food and Drug Administration (FDA): It is a regulatory authority that ensures food and medical products are of good quality and safe for human use.
Good practices: These are the techniques which when followed consistently show results that are superior to those achieved when these practices are not followed. Example - handwashing practices to prevent infections.
Hand care: It is the action to prevent skin irritation that may be caused by use of chemical agents for hand washing purpose.
Hand hygiene: Action of hand antisepsis in hygienic way so as to reduce transient microbial flora. This can be achieved either by hand washing with soap and water or by hand rubbing with alcohol-based formulation.
Hazards: Any phenomenon which has the potential to cause damage to population and environment from the extremes of natural process or manmade technologies.
Health screening: Process through which a series of tests are done in order to look for diseases before their symptoms develops. Screening helps in treating disease early as they are easier. Some screening need special equipments like mammography, bone densitometer, etc.
High level disinfection: Process that destroy vegetative bacteria, mycobacteria, fungi and enveloped (lipid) and nonenveloped (nonlipid) viruses but not necessarily bacterial spores. Thorough cleaning is prerequisite prior to high level disinfection. High level disinfectant chemicals are also called chemical sterilants.

Hospital associated infection: Also called nosocomial infection. These are the infections which affected patient or hospital staff as a consequence of working in hospital.

Immunology: The study of immunity and an individuals response to antigens.

Immunosuppressive drug: A drug that is administered to reduce the tendency of the living organism to reject tissues or an organ, e.g. kidney or heart from a donor.

Immunotherapy: The stimulation of the body's immune system as a means of treating cancer.

Incidence: It is the number of new cases of a disease occurring in a specific time.

Incidence rate: It is the ratio of number of new infections or diseases in a defined population in a given period to the number of individuals at risk in the population.

Incubation period: It is the time period which elapses between invasion of the body tissues by pathogens and appearance of first clinical symptoms and signs of infections.

Indicators: These are the variables which help in measuring the changes indirectly or directly so as to assess the extent to which the objectives are being achieved.

Infection: It is the deposition and multiplication of micro-organisms on the surfaces or in the tissues of the body with an associated tissue reaction. In case the response of host is minimal or absent then term colonization is used.

Infusion: The term applied to the injection of a solution into blood vessels or tissue underlying the skin.

Ingestion: Swallowing, by the oral route.

Inhalation: Breathing in.

Intended purpose: The use for which the device is intended according to the information supplied by the manufacturer on the label, in the instructions and/or promotional materials.

Intermediate level disinfection: This process kill vegetative bacteria, most of viruses and fungi but not resistant bacterial spores.

Invasive medical device: Any medical device which enter body through either a body opening or breaking mucous membrane or skin.

Irritant: A substance that will produce local irritation or inflammation on contact with tissues and membranes such as skin or eyes, or will, after inhalation, produce local irritation to nasal or lung tissue.

Isolation: Physical separation of infected host from the remainder of at the risk population in an attempt to prevent transmission of the specific agent to other individuals and to patients.
Laminar flow: An essentially unidirectional airflow with minimum turbulence.
Log book: A systematically arranged document which is marked with the time of action or event of substantial significance.
Low level disinfection: This process kill most of vegetative bacteria, some of fungi and enveloped (lipid) viruses like HIV, HBV, HCV. However these processes don't kill mycobacteria or bacterial spores. LLD is method of choice to clean environmental surfaces.
Medical devices: Any instrument, appliance, material or other article which is used alone or in combination intended by manufacturer to be used for human beings for the purpose for patient care either in the form of diagnostics or treatment.
Medical waste: Also known as clinical waste in the waste products which can not be considered as general waste and generated from healthcare settings.
Metabolite: In physiology, any product yielded by or taking part in the chemical processes essential to life.
Micro-organisms: The organism that can be seen only with the help of magnification of microscope. As used in health care, generally refers to bacteria, fungi, viruses, and bacterial spores.
Monitoring: It is the daily activity of management and consist of keeping track of course of activities and identify any deviation so that activities can be put back on their right track. It is also oversee the proceedings of activities going on as planned and are on scheduled.
Mutagenic: Able to cause mutations. Capable of causing alterations/damage to genes.
Needle stick injury: Percutaneous piercing wound caused by needle point or any other sharp medical device. This is a type of occupational hazard and are of concern because of transmission of blood borne diseases like HBV, HCV, HIV. This is a preventable occurrence if proper precautions are taken by the medical community.
Negative pressure room: It is single occupancy patient care room used mainly for isolation in case of suspected or confirmed air borne infectious disease. The care area's environmental factors are controlled to minimize transmission of infectious agents through droplet nuclei.
Neoplasm: Another word for tumor.

Noncritical items: Those items which come in contact with only intact skin but not mucous membrane or do not directly contact the patient. These items are reprocessed by cleaning followed by low level disinfection.
Notifiable diseases: These are diseases which are required by law to be notified to the public health authorities. Notifiable disease may vary from state to state but in common they are—malaria, dengue, viral hepatitis, TB, leptospirosis, polio, influenza, rabies, HIV/AIDS, leprosy, louse borne typhus.
Oncogenic: Causing or encouraging the growth of tumors.
Oncology: The science of new growth. It is that part of medical science which is concerned with the management of malignant disease such as cancer.
Outbreak: Presence of two or more epidemiological related cases of infection linked in place or time and all are caused by same micro-organism.
Parts per million: The common measurement used in concentration by volume of trace contaminant gases in the air or chemicals in liquids.
Personal protective equipments: This is type of barrier used alone or in combination to protect clothing, skin, mucous membranes from contact with infectious agents.
Precaution: An action which is taken in advance so as to protect against any possible injury, failure or danger. Example—take precautions while handling syringes to prevent NSI.
Prevalence rate: The ratio of the total number of individuals who have disease at a particular time to the population at risk of having the disease. It can be defined also as the number of cases of disease present in defined population at one point of risk.
Prevention: In medical literature context it means promotion of health, preservation and restoration of health when it is impaired and also reduce distress and sufferings.
Procedure: An act of patient care which is associated with a risk of direct introduction of a pathogen to the patient.
Process: It is a set of interrelated activities which transforms inputs into outputs.
Program: A sequence of activities designed to implement policies and achieve desired predetermined objectives.
Quality assurance: It is the part of quality management process with special focus on providing confidence to service users that quality requirements will be fulfilled.

Quality control: Mostly written as QC. It is consists of set of procedures which are collectively intended to ensure that the service provided adheres to a defined set of quality criteria or meet the requirements of the patients and their families.
Quarantine: It is a period of time during with a person or vehicle is suspected of carrying a transmissible, infectious or contagious disease detained at the port of entry under enforced isolation so as to prevent disease from entering the country.
Reprocessing: It is the process of subjecting the medical device to additional processing for the purpose of additional use of same device on a patient.
Reuse: Another episode or repeated episodes of use of medical device that has undergone some form of reprocessing between each episode.
Risk: It is the probability or threat of quantifiable damage, loss, injury or liability or any other negative occurrence which will be caused by internal or external vulnerabilities but are preventable if preemptive actions are taken.
Risk assessment: It is the part of risk management process. It determines qualitative as well as quantitative value of risk related to a situation and recognized threat in any organization.
Risk management in HCO: Collectively administrative and clinical activities in order to identify, evaluate, and reduce the risk of injury to care users as well as caregivers.
Sanitation: Process which reduces micro-organisms on an inanimate object to a level below which there is no infection hazard. For example eating in plates and utensils are sanitized.
Semicritical items: Those devices which come in contact with nonintact skin or mucous membrane but do not penetrate them. The reprocessing of these items includes meticulous cleaning followed by high level or intermediate level disinfection.
Sepsis: The presence of pus or acute inflammation in a wound.
Seroconversion: It is the acquisition for antibodies that may occur through infection or vaccination.
Sewage: Waste water that usually includes excreta which is or will be or has been carried in water.
Sharp containers: These are the puncture proof containers which are used to dispose off used needles or other sharps during patient care. The sharp need to be dropped in to the container they are neither forced or pushed in container as this act will either damage container or cause needle stick injury to the user.

Sharps: These are the instrument which are used in healthcare delivery and while doing to can inflict a penetrating injury like lancets, needles, scalpels, etc.

Single use device: It means that particular medical device is intended to be used on an individual patient during single procedure and then discarded.

Source: It is the place, person or thing from which the infectious agent spared to the host.

Spores: These are round or elliptical resting cells having condensed cytoplasm and nucleus secured by water proof wall or coat. Spores are relatively resistant to process of disinfection and drying conditions.

Standard operating procedures (SOPs): These are applicable to all employees of the organization. These contains detailed step by step explanation of how a policy is to be implemented. The SOP gives details about the task which is to be performed, i.e. who will do, when task is to be done, how it is to be done, what resources needed, where task is to be executed. The SOP acts as instructional resource which allows staff to perform the task without asking for direction, reassurance or guidance. Once the SOP is understood by staff they can be held accountable for any deviation from the standard.

Standard precautions: These are work practices which constitute first line approach to infection prevention and control while providing patient care in healthcare organization.

Sterile: It is the state of being free from all living microorganisms. This in usual practice described as a probability functions as the probability of micro-organisms surviving sterilization process being one in one million.

Sterilizer: Machines which are used to make patient care items undergo the process of sterilization.

Sterilizer gravity-displacement type: Sterilizing machine in which the incoming steam displaces residual air from the sterilizer chamber through a given port near the bottom.

Sterilizer prevacuum type: Sterilizing machine which depends on vacuum excursions at the start of cycle so as to remove air from sterilizer chamber. This methodology has shorter cycle time because of rapid removal of air from chamber and high operating temperature.

Sterilization: It is the process by which an object is made free from all viable micro-organisms including spores.

Strategies: Derived from the Greek word *strategia* it is the high level plan to achieve desired goal under conditions of uncertainty and limited resources.

Surgical site infection (SSI): Infection which occurs after surgical procedure at the site where the surgery took place. It may be superficial involving skin only or very serious life-threatening.
Surveillance: It is ongoing systemic and active observation of the occurrence and distribution of infections within a population, and also of the events the decreases or increases the risk of such infections. It is necessarily a multidisciplinary team effort.
Teratogenic: Able to produce abnormalities in a developing embryo or fetus, that is, causing birth defects.
Training: It is the acquisition of knowledge, skills and competencies as a result of teaching by trainer and will relate to specific and useful tasks.
Transmission: It is the indirect or direct transfer of disease from reservoir or source of infection to susceptible host.
Tumor: A swelling, enlargement, or an abnormal mass of tissue in which the growth of cells is uncontrolled. A tumor can either be benign (not malignant) or malignant (cancerous).
Universal precautions: Practices followed during patient care, to avoid contact with patients blood or body fluid, by wearing of non-porous articles like gloves, mask, apron, goggles, etc. now these are replaced by standard precautions in healthcare.
UTI: Infection of urinary tract and one of the most common cause of hospital acquired infection. It is mainly caused by *E. coli*.
Vaccination: It is the administration of weakened or live infectious organisms or their part or products to prevent the disease.
Validation: It is the documented procedure of obtaining and interpreting results required to establish that the said process will consistently yield a product complying with preset specifications.
Vegetative bacteria: These are the bacteria which are devoid of spores and can be easily and readily inactivated by various types of germicides. Bacteria that are devoid of spores and usually can be readily inactivated by many types of germicides.
Ventilator-associated pneumonia (VAP): Which develop within 48 hours of in person who has device to control or assist respiration continuously through either endotrachal tube or tracheostomy.
Virulence: It is the degree of pathogenicity of micro-organism as indicated by case fatality rate and/or ability of the organism to invade the tissues of the host.
Waste: It is the discarded material much of which can be reused or recycled or generate fertilizer by compositing such discarded material.
Waste audit: It is a methodical examination of all of the regulated biomedical waste at different stages of management as per rules.

It is done to ensure quality control and best practice standards at work place. Audit performed at final treatment and disposal site like autoclaving and incineration will be able to detect the fault with segregation, collection and transport. With the help of waste audit one can evaluate each step of the biomedical waste management.

Waste labeling: It is the process of coding with standards and well recognized international symbols and color make easy in the correct identification and safe management of medical waste. The process of labeling makes easy to understand the different categories of waste and give caution to all workers, visitors, family members patients and public about the existence of the waste.

Waste minimization: It is the application of activities which will eventually reduce the quantum of waste generation. Activities like reuse, recycling, reduce may be used to achieve minimization goal.

Waste segregation: It is the process of keeping biomedical waste separated from other waste during the process of handling, collection, storage and transport and ensure proper treatment and/or disposal are utilized.

WHO: World Health Organization (established on 7th April 1948) is a specialized agency of the United Nations which is concerned with international public health.

Annexures

Annexure A:
Checklist for Infection Control Measures

Date _____ Time _____ Name of inspector _____

1. Decontamination of instruments:
   a. Is sterilizer available   Yes/No
   b. Is it in good working condition   Yes/No
   c. Are clean instruments stored in cupboard under lock   Yes/No
   d. Are instruments rust free   Yes/No
2. Handling of sharp:
   a. Is puncture proof container available   Yes/No
   b. Are sharps popping out of containers   Yes/No
   c. Is sharp lying outside containers   Yes/No
   d. Is there any recapping of needles/syringes   Yes/No
   e. Is needle cutter available   Yes/No
   f. Is it in good working condition   Yes/No
3. Close of protective barrier:
   a. Are protective barriers available   Yes/No
   b. Are they in good condition   Yes/No
   c. Are they of good quality   Yes/No
   d. Are they being used by staff having the risk of exposure   Yes/No
4. Hand washing practices:
   a. Is soap and running clean water available   Yes/No
   b. Is paper towel/clean towel available   Yes/No
   c. Is staff aware of hand washing practices   Yes/No
   d. Are staff members washing their hands properly   Yes/No
5. Waste management:
   a. Is waste being managed as per rules   Yes/No
   b. Is there any contaminated waste littered around   Yes/No
   c. Are the container in good condition   Yes/No
   d. Does staff handle the waste with bare hands   Yes/No
   e. Are containers color coded as per rules   Yes/No

Annexure B:
Checklist for Maintenance of Incinerator

Day _____ Time _____ Name of inspector _____

1.	Is surrounding of incinerator is clean	Yes/No
2.	What is temp of primary chamber	..........°C
3.	What is temp of secondary chamber	..........°C
4.	Is auto switch off system working	Yes/No
5.	What is condition of primary chamber lining intact/broken	
6.	Loading of primary chamber optimum/under loading /over loading	
7.	Is record book of waste incinerator is available	Yes/No
8.	Is this record maintained up to date	Yes/No
9.	Has medical examination of incinerator staff is being done periodically	Yes/No
10.	Is such record of Medical Examination available	Yes/No
11.	Is incinerator ash is being disposed off as per rule	Yes/No
12.	Is APCU working properly	Yes/No
13.	What is color of smoke from stake black/white	
14.	Is record of maintenance of incinerator available	Yes/No
15.	How is the surrounding of incinerator clean/unclean	

Comment of Inspector _____

Signature

Annexure C:
Checklist for Biomedical Waste Management Audit

1.	Does the occupier has authority to set up its own treatment facility or having any other alternative option	Yes/No
2.	Is the segregation of waste is being done at the point of generation	Yes/No
3.	Is BMW mixed with other general waste	Yes/No
4.	Are waste collection containers available	Yes/No
5.	Are containers color coded as per the rule	Yes/No
6.	Does the waste marked for incineration have plastic waste mixed in it	Yes/No
7.	Does the institution has system for waste classification	Yes/No
8.	Are the containers in good condition	Yes/No
9.	Is institution taking steps for BMWM as per the category and recommended method of treatment and disposal for that particular category	Yes/No
10.	Is spill treatment kit available	Yes/No
11.	Is institution having SOP for mercury spill management	Yes/No
12.	Is liquid waste being treated with 1% hypochlorite solution before discharge into sewers	Yes/No
13.	Are needle destroyer available in sufficient number	Yes/No
14.	Are needle destroyer in good working condition	Yes/No
15.	Is there proper storage and internal and external transport facility available	Yes/No
16.	Are these facilities as per BMWM rule 1998	Yes/No
17.	Do employees wear protective barrier while on the job	Yes/No
18.	Is there any incidence of occupational injury	Yes/No
19.	Is the record of such injury along with phone number is available	Yes/No
20.	Is record of every day's generation of waste is available as per the category	Yes/No
21.	Is there any accessibility of unauthorized person to waste storage	Yes/No
22.	Is separate facility for treated and untreated waste storage is available	Yes/No
23.	In case Institution is using CBTF, then is record of agreement available	Yes/No
24.	Is there any separate route for waste transport	Yes/No
25.	Is institution having recorded policy on the waste type, collection time and weighing of waste	Yes/No
26.	Is medical examination record of waste handlers available	Yes/No

27. Is the vehicle, which is carrying waste from institution to off site authorized for such specialized work Yes/No
28. Is training manual for staff available Yes/No
29. Is record of employees training available Yes/No
30. Are colored plastic bags in good condition Yes/No
31. Is waste generator aware of difference between soiled and unsoiled waste Yes/No

Annexure D:
Forms as per the Gazette of India
Ministry of Environment of Forest, New Delhi, 20th July 1998

FORM I
Notice of Intention to have Sample Analyzed

To

....

....

Take notice that it is intended to have analysed the sample of .... which has been taken today, the day of 19 from (Name and designation of the person who takes the sample) Specify the place from where the sample is taken.

(Seal)

Date: ....

FORM II
Memorandum to Government Analyst

From

....

....

To

The Government Analyst

....

....

The portion of sample described below is sent herewith for analysis under rule 6 of the Environment (Protection) Rules, 1986. The portion of the sample has been marked by me with the following mark. Details of the portion of sample taken.

Name and designation of
Person who sends sample
(Seal)

Date: ....

FORM III
Report by Government Analyst

Report No. ....

Date: ....

    I hereby certify that I .... Government Analyst duly appointed under section 13 of the Environment (Protection) Act, 1986 received on the .... day of .... from .... a sample of .... for analysis.

    The sample was in a condition fit for analysis as reported below.

    I further certify that I have analyzed the above mentioned sample on ... . and declare the result of the analysis to be as follows:

** ....
. ...

    The condition of seals fastening of sample on receipt was as follows: ....

    Signed this...day of........................19..............
..

    Address..

Signature
(Government Analyst)

To

....
....
....

    Here write the name of the officer/authority from whom sample was obtained.

    **Here write full details of analysis and refer to method of analysis.

FORM IV
Form of Notice

By registered post acknowledgement due

Form (1)

Shri ....

....

....

To

....

....

Notice Under Section 19(b) of the Environment (Protection) Act, 1986 whereas an offence under the Environment (Protection) Act, 1986 has been committed/is being committed by .... (1) I/We hereby give notice of 60 days under Section 19(b) of the Environment (Protection) Act, 1986 of my/our intention to file a complaint in the court against .... (2) for violation of Section of the Environment (Protection) Act, 1986.

In support of my/our notice, I am/we are enclosing the following documents (3) as evidence of proof of violation of the Environment (Protection) Act, 1986.

Place: ....   Signature (s)

Dated: ....

Explanation:
1. In case the notice is given in the name of a company, documentary evidence authorizing the person to sign the notice on behalf of the company shall be enclosed to this notice.
   Company for this purpose means a company defined in explanation to subrule (6) of rule 4.
2. Here given the name and address of the alleged offender. In case of a manufacturing /processing /operating unit, indicate in the name/location/nature of activity, etc.
3. Documentary evidence shall include photographs/technical reports/health reports of the area, etc. for enabling enquiry into the alleged violation/offence.

Annexure E:
Schedules of BMW (Handling and Management) Rules, 2016

SCHEDULE I
[See rules 3 (e), 4(b), 7(1), 7(2), 7(5), 7 (6) and 8(2)]

PART-1

Biomedical wastes categories and their segregation, collection, treatment, processing and disposal options:

Category	Type of waste	Type of bag or container to be used	Treatment and disposal options
(1)	(2)	(3)	(4)
Yellow	(a) **Human anatomical waste:** Human tissues, organs, body parts and fetus below the viability period (as per the Medical Termination of Pregnancy Act 1971, amended from time to time).	Yellow colored non-chlorinated plastic bags	Incineration or plasma pyrolysis or deep burial*
	(b) **Animal anatomical waste:** Experimental animal carcasses, body parts, organs, tissues, including the waste generated from animals used in experiments or testing in veterinary hospitals or colleges or animal houses.		
	(c) **Soiled waste:** Items contaminated with blood, body fluids like dressings, plaster casts, cotton		Incineration or plasma pyrolysis or deep burial* In absence of above facilities,

Contd...

Contd...

Category (1)	Type of waste (2)	Type of bag or container to be used (3)	Treatment and disposal options (4)
	swabs and bags containing residual or discarded blood and blood components.		autoclaving or micro-waving/ hydroclaving followed by shredding or mutilation or combination of sterilization and shredding. Treated waste to be sent for energy recovery.
	(d) Expired or discarded medicines: Pharmaceutical waste like antibiotics, cytotoxic drugs including all items contaminated with cytotoxic drugs along with glass or plastic ampoules, vials etc.	Yellow colored non-chlorinated plastic bags or containers	Expired 'cytotoxic drugs and items contaminated with cytotoxic drugs to be returned back to the manufacturer or supplier for incineration at temperature >1200°C or to common bio-medical waste treatment facility or hazardous waste treatment, storage and disposal facility for incineration at >1200°C or encapsulation or plasma pyrolysis at >1200°C. All other discarded medicines shall be either sent back to manufacturer or disposed by incineration.

Contd...

Contd...

Category (1)	Type of waste (2)	Type of bag or container to be used (3)	Treatment and disposal options (4)
	(e) Chemical waste: Chemicals used in production of biological and used or discarded disinfectants.	Yellow colored containers or non-chlorinated plastic bags	Disposed of by incineration or plasma pyrolysis or encapsulation in hazardous waste treatment, storage and disposal facility.
	(f) Chemical liquid waste: Liquid waste generated due to use of chemicals in production of biological and used or discarded disinfectants, silver X-ray film developing liquid, discarded formalin, infected secretions, aspirated body fluids, liquid from laboratories and floor washings, cleaning, house-keeping and disinfecting activities etc.	Separate collection system leading to effluent treatment system	After resource recovery, the chemical liquid waste shall be pre-treated before mixing with other wastewater. The combined discharge shall conform to the discharge norms given in Schedule-III.
	(g) Discarded linen, mattresses, beddings contaminated with blood or body fluid.	Non-chlorinated yellow plastic bags or suitable packing material	Non-chlorinated chemical disinfection followed by incineration or plazma pyrolysis or for energy recovery. In absence of above facilities, shredding or mutilation or

Contd...

Contd...

Category (1)	Type of waste (2)	Type of bag or container to be used (3)	Treatment and disposal options (4)
			combination of sterilization and shredding. Treated waste to be sent for energy recovery or incineration or plazma pyrolysis.
	(h) Microbiology, biotechnology and other clinical laboratory waste: Blood bags, laboratory cultures, stocks or specimens of micro-organisms, live or attenuated vaccines, human and animal cell cultures used in research, industrial laboratories, production of biological, residual toxins, dishes and devices used for cultures.	Autoclave safe plastic bags or containers	Pre-treat to sterilize with non-chlorinated chemicals on-site as per National AIDS Control Organisation or World Health Organisation guidelines thereafter for Incineration.
Red	**Contaminated waste (recyclable):** Wastes generated from disposable items such as tubing, bottles, intravenous tubes and sets, catheters, urine bags, syringes (without needles and *fixed needle syringes*) and vaccutainers with their needles cut) and gloves.	Red colored non-chlorinated plastic bags or containers	Autoclaving or micro-waving/ hydroclaving followed by shredding or mutilation or combination of sterilization and shredding. Treated waste to be sent to registered or authorized recyclers or for energy recovery or

Contd...

Contd...

Category (1)	Type of waste (2)	Type of bag or container to be used (3)	Treatment and disposal options (4)
			plastics to diesel or fuel oil or for road making, whichever is possible. Plastic waste should not be sent to landfill sites.
White (translucent)	**Waste sharps including metals:** Needles, syringes with fixed needles, needles from needle tip cutter or burner, scalpels, blades, or any other contaminated sharp object that may cause puncture and cuts. This includes both used, discarded and contaminated metal sharps	Puncture proof, leak proof, tamper proof containers	Autoclaving or dry heat sterilization followed by shredding or mutilation or encapsulation in metal container or cement concrete; combination of shredding cum autoclaving; and sent for final disposal to iron foundries (having consent to operate from the State Pollution Control Boards or Pollution Control Committees) or sanitary landfill or designated concrete waste sharp pit.
Blue	**(a) Glassware:** Broken or discarded and contaminated glass including medicine vials and ampoules except those contaminated with cytotoxic wastes.	Cardboard boxes with blue colored marking	Disinfection (by soaking the washed glass waste after cleaning with detergent and sodium hypochlorite treatment)

Contd...

Contd...

Category (1)	Type of waste (2)	Type of bag or container to be used (3)	Treatment and disposal options (4)
			or through autoclaving or microwaving or hydroclaving and then sent for recycling.
	(b) Metallic body implants	Cardboard boxes with blue colored marking	

*Disposal by deep burial is permitted only in rural or remote areas where there is no access to common bio-medical waste treatment facility. This will be carried out with prior approval from the prescribed authority and as per the Standards specified in Schedule-III. The deep burial facility shall be located as per the provisions and guidelines issued by Central Pollution Control Board from time to **time.**

PART -2

1. All plastic bags shall be as per BIS standards as and when published, till then the prevailing Plastic Waste Management Rules shall be applicable.
2. Chemical treatment using at least 10% Sodium Hypochlorite having 30% residual chlorine for 20 minutes or any other equivalent chemical reagent that should demonstrate $Log_{10}4$ reduction efficiency for microorganisms as given in Schedule- III.
3. Mutilation or shredding must be to an extent to prevent unauthorized reuse.
4. There will be no chemical pretreatment before incineration, except for microbiological, lab and highly infectious waste.
5. Incineration ash (ash from incineration of any bio-medical waste) shall be disposed through hazardous waste treatment, storage and disposal facility, if toxic or hazardous constituents are present beyond the prescribed limits as given in the Hazardous Waste (Management, Handling and Transboundary Movement) Rules, 2008 or as revised from time to time.
6. Dead Fetus below the viability period (as per the Medical Termination of Pregnancy Act 1971, amended from time to time) can be considered

as human anatomical waste. Such waste should be handed over to the operator of common bio-medical waste treatment and disposal facility in yellow bag with a copy of the official Medical Termination of Pregnancy certificate from the Obstetrician or the Medical Superintendent of hospital or healthcare establishment.

7. Cytotoxic drug vials shall not be handed over to unauthorised person under any circumstances. These shall be sent back to the manufactures for necessary disposal at a single point. As a second option, these may be sent for incineration at common bio-medical waste treatment and disposal facility or TSDFs or plasma pyrolys is at temperature >1200°C.

8. Residual or discarded chemical wastes, used or discarded disinfectants and chemical sludge can be disposed at hazardous waste treatment, storage and disposal facility. In such case, the waste should be sent to hazardous waste treatment, storage and disposal facility through operator of common bio-medical waste treatment and disposal facility only.

9. On-site pre-treatment of laboratory waste, microbiological waste, blood samples, blood bags should be disinfected or sterilized as per the Guidelines of World Health Organisation or National AIDS Control Organisation and then given to the common bio-medical waste treatment and disposal facility.

10. Installation of in-house incinerator is not allowed. However in case there is no common biomedical facility nearby, the same may be installed by the occupier after taking authorisation from the State Pollution Control Board.

11. Syringes should be either mutilated or needles should be cut and or stored in tamper proof, leak proof and puncture proof containers for sharps storage. Wherever the occupier is not linked to a disposal facility it shall be the responsibility of the occupier to sterilize and dispose in the manner prescribed.

12. Bio-medical waste generated in households during healthcare activities shall be segregated as per these rules and handed over in separate bags or containers to municipal waste collectors. Urban Local Bodies shall have tie up with the common bio-medical waste treatment and disposal facility to pickup this waste from the Material Recovery Facility (MRF) or from the household directly, for final disposal in the manner as prescribed in this Schedule.

SCHEDULE II
[See rule 4(t), 7(1) and 7(6)]
STANDARDS FOR TREATMENT AND DISPOSAL OF BIO-MEDICALWASTES

1. STANDARDS FOR INCINERATION.-
All incinerators shall meet the following operating and emission standards:

A. Operating Standards
1. Combustion efficiency (CE) shall be at least 99.00%.
2. The combustion efficiency is computed as follows:
$$CE = \frac{\%CO_2}{\%CO_2 + \%CO} \times 100$$
3. The temperature of the primary chamber shall be a minimum of 800°C and the secondary chamber shall be minimum of 1050°C + or –50°C.
4. The secondary chamber gas residence time shall be at least two seconds.

B. Emission Standards

Sl. No.	Parameter	Standards	
(1)	(2)	(3)	(4)
		Limiting concentration in mg Nm^3 unless stated	Sampling duration in minutes, unless stated
1.	Particulate matter	50	30 or 1 NM^3 of sample volume, whichever is more
2.	Nitrogen Oxides NO and NO_2 expressed as NO_2	400	30 for online sampling or grab sample
3.	HCl	50	30 or 1 NM^3 of sample volume, whichever is more
4.	Total Dioxins and Furans	0.1ngTEQ/Nm^3 (at 11% O_2)	8 hours or 5 NM^3 of sample volume, whichever is more
5.	Hg and its compounds	0.05	2 hours or 1 NM^3 of sample volume, whichever is more

C. Stack Height: Minimum stack height shall be 30 meters above the ground and shall be attached with the necessary monitoring facilities as per requirement of monitoring of 'general parameters' as notified under the

Environment (Protection) Act, 1986 and in accordance with the Central Pollution Control Board Guidelines of Emission Regulation Part-III.

Note:
a. The existing incinerators shall comply with the above within a period of two years from the date of the notification.
b. The existing incinerators shall comply with the standards for Dioxins and Furans of 0.1ngTEQ/Nm^3, as given below within two years from the date of commencement of these rules.
c. All upcoming common bio-medical waste treatment facilities having incineration facility or captive incinerator shall comply with standards for Dioxins and Furans.
d. The existing secondary combustion chambers of the incinerator and the pollution control devices shall be suitably retrofitted, if necessary, to achieve the emission limits.
e. Wastes to be incinerated shall not be chemically treated with any chlorinated disinfectants.
f. Ash from incineration of biomedical waste shall be disposed of at common hazardous waste treatment and disposal facility. However, it may be disposed of in municipal landfill, if the toxic metals in incineration ash are within the regulatory quantities as defined under the Hazardous Waste (Management and Handling and Transboundary Movement) Rules, 2008 as amended from time to time.
g. Only low Sulphur fuel like Light Diesel Oil or Low Sulphur Heavy Stock or Diesel, Compressed Natural Gas, Liquefied Natural Gas or Liquefied Petroleum Gas shall be used as fuel in the incinerator.
h. The occupier or operator of a common bio-medical waste treatment facility shall monitor the stack gaseous emissions (under optimum capacity of the incinerator) once in three months through a laboratory approved under the Environment (Protection) Act, 1986 and record of such analysis results shall be maintained and submitted to the prescribed authority. In case of dioxins and furans, monitoring should be done once in a year.
i. The occupier or operator of the common bio-medical waste treatment facility shall install continuous emission monitoring system for the parameters as stipulated by State Pollution Control Board or Pollution Control Committees in authorisation and transmit the data real time to the servers at State Pollution Control Board or Pollution Control Committees and Central Pollution Control Board.
j. All monitored values shall be corrected to 11% oxygen on dry basis.
k. Incinerators (combustion chambers) shall be operated with such temperature, retention time and turbulence, as to achieve total organic carbon content in the slag and bottom ashes less than 3% or their loss on ignition shall be less than 5% of the dry weight.
l. The occupier or operator of a common bio-medical waste incinerator shall use combustion gas analyzer to measure CO_2, CO and O_2.

2. OPERATING AND EMISSION STANDARDS FOR DISPOSAL BY PLASMA PYROLYSIS OR GASIFICATION:

A. Operating Standards

All the operators of the Plasma Pyrolysis or Gasification shall meet the following operating and emission standards:
1. Combustion efficiency (CE) shall be at least 99.99%.
2. The combustion efficiency is computed as follows:

$$CE = \frac{\%CO_2}{\%CO_2 + \%CO} \times 100$$

3. The temperature of the combustion chamber after plasma gasification shall be 1050 ± 50°C with gas residence time of at least 2(two) second, with minimum 3 % oxygen in the stack gas.
4. The stack height should be minimum of 30 m above ground level and shall be attached with the necessary monitoring facilities as per requirement of monitoring of 'general parameters' as notified under the Environment (Protection) Act, 1986 and in accordance with the CPCB Guidelines of Emission Regulation Part-III.

B. Air Emission Standards and Air Pollution Control Measures
1. Emission standards for incinerator, notified at Sl. No.1 above in this Schedule, and revised from time to time, shall be applicable for the plasma pyrolysis or gasification also.
2. Suitably designed air pollution control devices shall be installed or retrofitted with the 'plasma pyrolysis or gasification to achieve the above emission limits, if necessary.
3. Wastes to be treated using plasma pyrolysis or gasification shall not be chemically treated with any chlorinated disinfectants and chlorinated plastics shall not be treated in the system.

C. Disposal of Ash Vitrified Material: The ash or vitrified material generated from the 'Plasma Pyrolysis or Gasification shall be disposed off in accordance with the Hazardous Waste (Management, Handling and Transboundary Movement) Rules 2008 and revisions made thereafter in case the constituents exceed the limits prescribed under Schedule II of the said Rules or else in accordance with the provisions of the Environment (Protection) Act, 1986, whichever is applicable.

3. STANDARDS FOR AUTOCLAVING OF BIO-MEDICAL WASTE:

The autoclave should be dedicated for the purposes of disinfecting and treating bio-medical waste.
1. When operating a gravity flow autoclave, medical waste shall be subjected to:
    i. A temperature of not less than 121° C and pressure of 15 pounds per square inch (psi) for an autoclave residence time of not less than 60 minutes; or
    ii. A temperature of not less than 135° C and a pressure of 31 psi for an autoclave residence time of not less than 45 minutes; or

      iii. A temperature of not less than 149° C and a pressure of 52 psi for an autoclave residence time of not less than 30 minutes.
2. When operating a vacuum autoclave, medical waste shall be subjected to a minimum of three pre-vacuum pulse to purge the autoclave of all air. The air removed during the pre-vacuum, cycle should be decontaminated by means of HEPA and activated carbon filtration, steam treatment, or any other method to prevent release of pathogen. The waste shall be subjected to the following:
    i. A temperature of not less than 121°C and pressure of 15 psi per an autoclave residence time of not less than 45 minutes; or
    ii. A temperature of not less than 135°C and a pressure of 31 psi for an autoclave residence time of not less than 30 minutes;
3. Medical waste shall not be considered as properly treated unless the time, temperature and pressure indicators indicate that the required time, temperature and pressure were reached during the autoclave process. If for any reasons, time temperature or pressure indicator indicates that the required temperature, pressure or residence time was not reached, the entire load of medical waste must be autoclaved again until the proper temperature, pressure and residence time were achieved.
4. **Recording of operational parameters:** Each autoclave shall have graphic or computer recording devices which will automatically and continuously monitor and record dates, time of day, load identification number and operating parameters throughout the entire length of the autoclave cycle.
5. **Validation test for autoclave:** The validation test shall use four biological indicator strips, one shall be used as a control and left at room temperature, and three shall be placed in the approximate center of three containers with the waste. Personal protective equipment (gloves, face mask and coveralls) shall be used when opening containers for the purpose of placing the biological indicators. At least one of the containers with a biological indicator should be placed in the most difficult location for steam to penetrate, generally the bottom center of the waste pile. The occupier or operator shall conduct this test three consecutive times to define the minimum operating conditions. The temperature, pressure and residence time at which all biological indicator vials or strips for three consecutive tests show complete inactivation of the spores shall define the minimum operating conditions for the autoclave. After determining the minimum temperature, pressure and residence time, the occupier or operator of a common biomedical waste treatment facility shall conduct this test once in three months and records in this regard shall be maintained.
6. **Routine test:** A chemical indicator strip or tape that changes color when a certain temperature is reached can be used to verify that a specific temperature has been achieved. It may be necessary to use more than one strip over the waste package at different locations to ensure that

the inner content of the package has been adequately autoclaved. The occupier or operator of a common bio medical waste treatment facility shall conduct this test during autoclaving of each batch and records in this regard shall be maintained.

7. **Spore testing:** The autoclave should completely and consistently kill the approved biological indicator at the maximum design capacity of each autoclave unit. Biological indicator for autoclave shall be *Geobacillus stearothermophilus* spores using vials or spore strips; with at least 1×10^6 spores. Under no circumstances will an autoclave have minimum operating parameters less than a residence time of 30 minutes, a temperature less than 121°C or a pressure less than 15 psi. The occupier or operator of a common bio medical waste treatment and disposal facility shall conduct this test at least once in every week and records in this regard shall be maintained.

4. STANDARDS OF MICROWAVING:
1. Microwave treatment shall not be used for cytotoxic, hazardous or radioactive wastes, contaminated animal carcasses, body parts and large metal items.
2. The microwave system shall comply with the efficacy test or routine tests and a performance guarantee may be provided by the supplier before operation of the limit.
3. The microwave should completely and consistently kill the bacteria and other pathogenic organisms that are ensured by approved biological indicator at the maximum design capacity of each microwave unit. Biological indicators for microwave shall be *Bacillus atrophaeus* spores using vials or spore strips with at least 1×10^4 spores per detachable strip. The biological indicator shall be placed with waste and exposed to same conditions as the waste during a normal treatment cycle.

5. STANDARDS FOR DEEP BURIAL:
1. A pit or trench should be dug about two meters deep. It should be half filled with waste, then covered with lime within 50 cm of the surface, before filling the rest of the pit with soil.
2. It must be ensured that animals do not have any access to burial sites. Covers of galvanised iron or wire meshes may be used.
3. On each occasion, when wastes are added to the pit, a layer of 10 cm of soil shall be added to cover the wastes.
4. Burial must be performed under close and dedicated supervision.
5. The deep burial site should be relatively impermeable and no shallow well should be close to the site.
6. The pits should be distant from habitation, and located so as to ensure that no contamination occurs to surface water or ground water. The area should not be prone to flooding or erosion.
7. The location of the deep burial site shall be authorised by the prescribed authority.

8. The institution shall maintain a record of all pits used for deep burial.
9. The ground water table level should be a minimum of six meters below the lower level of deep burial pit.

6. STANDARDS FOR EFFICACY OF CHEMICAL DISINFECTION:

Microbial inactivation efficacy is equated to "Log10 kill" which is defined as the difference between the logarithms of number of test microorganisms before and after chemical treatment. Chemical disinfection methods shall demonstrate a 4 Log10 reduction or greater for Bacillus Subtilis (ATCC 19659) in chemical treatment systems.

7. STANDARDS FOR DRY HEAT STERILIZATION:

Waste sharps can be treated by dry heat sterilization at a temperature not less than 185°C, at least for a residence period of 150 minutes in each cycle, which sterilization period of 90 minutes. There should be automatic recording system to monitor operating parameters.

1. **Validation test for shaprs sterilization unit:** Waste shaprs sterilization unit should completely and consistently kill the biological indicator *Geobacillus stearothermophillus* or *Bacillus atropheaus* spores using vials with at least $\log_{10}$ 6 spores per mL. The test shall be carried out once in three months
2. **Routine test:** A chemical indicator strip or tape that changes color when a certain temperature is reached can be used to verify that a specific temperature has been achieved. It may be necessary to use more than one strip over the waste to ensure that the inner content of the sharps has been adequately disinfected. This test shall be performed once in week and records in this regard shall be maintained.

8. STANDARDS FOR LIQUID WASTE:

1. The effluent generated or treated from the premises of occupier or operator of a common biomedical waste treatment and disposal facility, before discharge into the sewer should conform to the following limits:

Parameters	Permissible limits
pH	6.5-9.0
Suspended solids	100 mg/L
Oil and grease	10 mg/L
BOD	30 mg/L
COD	250 mg/L
Bio-assay test	90% survival of fish after 96 hours in 100% effluent.

2. Sludge from Effluent Treatment Plant shall be given to common bio-medical waste treatment facility for incineration or to hazardous waste treatment, storage and disposal facility for disposal.

SCHEDULE III
[See rule 6 and 9(3)]
List of Prescribed Authorities and the Corresponding Duties

Sl. No.	Authority	Corresponding Duties
(1)	(2)	(3)
1.	Ministry of Environment, Forest and Climate Change, Government of India	1. Making policies concerning bio-medical waste management in the country including notification of rules and amendments to the rules as and when required. 2. Providing financial assistance for training and awareness programs on bio-medical waste management related activities to for the State Pollution Control Boards or Pollution Control Committees. 3. Facilitating financial assistance for setting up or upgradation of common bio-medical waste treatment facilities. 4. Undertake or support operational research and assessment with reference to risks to environment and health due to bio-medical waste and previously unknown disposables and wastes from new types of equipment. 5. Constitution of monitoring committee for implementation of the rules. 6. Hearing appeals and give decision made in Form- V against order passed by the prescribed authorities. 7. Develop standard manual for trainers and training. 8. Notify the standards or operating parameters for new technologies for treatment of biomedical waste other than those listed in Schedule-I.
2.	Central or State Ministry of Health and Family Welfare, Central Ministry for Animal Husbandry and Veterinary or State Department of	1. Grant of license to healthcare facilities or nursing homes or veterinary establishments with a condition to obtain authorisation from the prescribed authority for bio-medical waste management.

Contd...

Contd...

Sl. No. (1)	Authority (2)	Corresponding Duties (3)
	Animal Husbandry and Veterinary	2. Monitoring, refusal or cancellation of license for healthcare facilities or nursing homes or veterinary establishments for violations of conditions of authorisation or provisions under these rules. 3. Publication of list of registered healthcare facilities with regard to bio-medical waste generation, treatment and disposal. 4. Undertake or support operational research and assessment with reference to risks to environment and health due to bio-medical waste and previously unknown disposables and wastes from new types of equipment. 5. Coordinate with State Pollution Control Boards for organizing training programmes to staff of health care facilities and municipal workers on bio-medical waste. 6. Constitution of Expert Committees at National or State level for overall review and promotion of clean or new technologies for bio-medical waste management. 7. Organizing or Sponsoring of trainings for the regulatory authorities and healthcare facilities on bio-medical waste management related activities. 8. Sponsoring of mass awareness campaigns in electronic media and print media.
3.	Ministry of Defence	1. Grant and renewal of authorisation to Armed Forces healthcare facilities or common bio-medical waste treatment facilities (Rule 9). 2. Conduct training courses for authorities dealing with management of bio-medical wastes in Armed Forces health-

Contd...

Contd...

Sl. No.	Authority	Corresponding Duties
(1)	(2)	(3)
		care facilities or treatment facilities in association with State Pollution Control Boards or Pollution Control Committees or Central Pollution Control Board or Ministry of Environment, Forest and Climate Change. 3. Publication of inventory of occupiers and bio- medical waste generation from Armed Forces healthcare facilities or occupiers 4. Constitution of Advisory Committee for implementation of the rules. 5. Review of management of bio-medical waste generation in the Armed Forces healthcare facilities through its Advisory Committee (Rule 11). 6. Submission of annual report to Central Pollution Control Board within the stipulated time period (Rule 13).
4.	Central Pollution Control Board	1. Prepare Guidelines on bio-medical waste Management and submit to the Ministry of Environment, Forest and Climate Change. 2. Co-ordination of activities of State Pollution Control Boards or Pollution Control Committees on bio- medical waste. 3. Conduct training courses for authorities dealing with management of bio-medical waste. 4. Lay down standards for new technologies for treatment and disposal of bio-medical waste (Rule 7) and prescribe specifications for treatment and disposal of bio-medical wastes (Rule 7). 5. Lay down Criteria for establishing common bio- medical waste treatment facilities in the Country.

Contd...

Contd...

Sl. No. (1)	Authority (2)	Corresponding Duties (3)
		6. Random inspection or monitoring of healthcare facilities and common bio-medical waste treatment facilities.
		7. Review and analysis of data submitted by the State Pollution Control Boards on bio-medical waste and submission of compiled information in the form of annual report along with its observations to Ministry of Environment, Forest and Climate Change.
		8. Inspection and monitoring of health care facilities operated by the Director General, Armed Forces Medical Services (Rule 9).
		9. Undertake or support research or operational research regarding bio-medical waste.
5.	State Government of Health or Union Territory Government or Administration	1. To ensure implementation of the rule in all healthcare facilities or occupiers.
		2. Allocation of adequate funds to Government healthcare facilities for bio-medical waste management.
		3. Procurement and allocation of treatment equipments and make provision for consumables for bio-medical waste management in Government health care facilities.
		4. Constitute State or District Level Advisory Committees under the District Magistrate or Additional District Magistrate to oversee the bio-medical waste management in the Districts.
		5. Advise State Pollution Control Boards or Pollution Control Committees on implementation of these Rules.
		6. Implementation of recommendations of the Advisory Committee in all the healthcare facilities.

Contd...

Contd...

Sl. No.	Authority	Corresponding Duties
(1)	(2)	(3)
6.	State Pollution Control Boards or Pollution Control Committees	1. Inventorisation of occupiers and data on bio-medical waste generation, treatment and disposal. 2. Compilation of data and submission of the same in annual report to Central Pollution Control Board within the stipulated time period. 3. Grant and renewal, suspension or refusal cancellation or of authorisation under these rules (Rule 7, 8 and 10). 4. Monitoring of compliance of various provisions and conditions of authorisation. 5. Action against healthcare facilities or common bio-medical waste treatment facilities for violation of these rules (Rule 18). 6. Organizing training programmes to staff of healthcare facilities and common bio-medical waste treatment facilities and State Pollution Control Boards or Pollution Control Committees Staff on segregation, collection, storage, transportation, treatment and disposal of bio-medical wastes. 7. Undertake or support research or operational research regarding bio-medical waste management. 8. Any other function under these rules assigned by Ministry of Environment, Forest and Climate Change or Central Pollution Control Board from time to time. 9. Implementation of recommendations of the Advisory Committee. 10. Publish the list of Registered or Authorised (or give consent) Recyclers. 11. Undertake and support third party audits of the common bio-medical waste treatment facilities in their State.

Contd...

Contd...

Sl. No.	Authority	Corresponding Duties
(1)	(2)	(3)
7.	Municipalities or Corporations, Urban Local Bodies and Gram Panchayats	1. Provide or allocate suitable land for development of common bio-medical waste treatment facilities in their respective jurisdictions as per the guidelines of Central Pollution Control Board. 2. Collect other solid waste (other than the bio- medical waste) from the health care facilities as per the Municipal Solid Waste (Management and handling) Rules, 2000 or as amended time to time. 3. Any other function stipulated under these Rules.

SCHEDULE IV
[See rule 8(3) and (5)]

PART A
Label for Biomedical Waste Container or Bags

Biohazard symbol   **Cytotoxic hazard symbol**

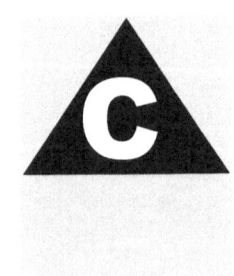

Handle with care   Handle with care

PART B
Label for Biomedical Waste Container or Bags

Day .... Month ....

Year ....

Date of generation ....

Waste category No. ....

Waste quantity ....

Sender's name and address   Receiver's name and address

Phone No. ....   Phone No. ....

Fax No. ....   Fax No. ....

Contact person ....   Contact person ....

In case of emergency, Please contact ....

Name and address ....

Phone No. ....

Note: Label shall be non-washable and prominently visible.

Annexure F:
Forms as per BMW (Handling and Management) Rules, 2016

FORM I
[(See rule 4(o), 5(i) and 15 (2)]
Accident Reporting

1. Date and time of accident :
2. Type of accident :
3. Sequence of events leading to accident :
4. Has the authority been informed immediately :
5. The type of waste involved in accident :
6. Assessment of the effects of the accidents on human health and the environment:
7. Emergency measures taken :
8. Steps taken to alleviate the effects of accidents :
9. Steps taken to prevent the recurrence of such an accident :
10. Does your facility has an Emergency Control policy? If yes give details:

Date ....   Signature ....

Place ....   Designation ....

FORM II
(See rule 10)
Application For Authorisation Or Renewal Of Authorisation
(To be submitted by occupier of healthcare facility or common bio-medical waste treatment facility)

To

The Prescribed Authority

(Name of the State or UT Administration) Address.

1. Particulars of Applicant:
    a. Name of the Applicant:
       (In block letters and in full)
    b. Name of the healthcare facility (HCF) or common bio-medical waste treatment facility (CBWTF):
    c. Address for correspondence:
    d. Tele No., Fax No.:
    e. Email:
    f. Website Address:
2. Activity for which authorisation is sought:

Activity	Please tick
Generation, segregation	
Collection,	
Storage packaging	
Reception	
Transportation	
Treatment or processing or conversion	
Recycling	
Disposal or destruction	
use	

offering for sale, transfer

Any other form of handling

3. Application for ☒ fresh or ☒ renewal of authorisation (please tick whatever is applicable):

   a. Applied for CTO/CTE Yes/No

   b. In case of renewal previous authorisation number and date:

   c. Status of Consents:

      i. Under the Water (Prevention and Control of Pollution) Act, 1974

      ii. Under the Air (Prevention and Control of Pollution) Act, 1981:

4. a. Address of the healthcare facility (HCF) or common bio-medical waste treatment facility (CBWTF):

   b. GPS coordinates of healthcare facility (HCF) or common bio-medical waste treatment facility (CBWTF):

5. Details of healthcare facility (HCF) or common bio-medical waste treatment facility (CBWTF):

   a. Number of beds of HCF:

   b. Number of patients treated per month by HCF:

   c. Number healthcare facilities covered by CBMWTF: _

   d. No of beds covered by CBMWTF: _____

   fe Installed treatment and disposal capacity of CBMWTF:_____ kg per day

   f. Quantity of biomedical waste treated or disposed by CBMWTF:_____kg/day

   g. Area or distance covered by CBMWTF:_____

   h. (pl. attach map a map with GPS locations of CBMWTF and area of coverage)

i. Quantity of biomedical waste handled, treated or disposed:

Category	Type of waste	Quantity generated or collected, kg/day	Method of treatment and disposal (Refer Schedule-I)
(1)	(2)	(3)	(4)
Yellow	a. Human anatomical waste:		
	b. Animal anatomical waste:		
	c. Soiled waste:		
	d. Expired or discarded medicines:		
	e. Chemical solid waste:		
	f. Chemical liquid waste:		
	g. Discarded linen, mattresses, beddings contaminated with blood or body fluid.		
	h. Microbiology, biotechnology and other clinical laboratory waste:		
Red	Contaminated waste (recyclable)		
White (translucent)	Waste sharps including metals:		
Blue	Glassware:		
	Metallic body implants		

6. Brief description of arrangements for handling of biomedical waste (attach details):

   a. Mode of transportation (if any) of bio-medical waste:

   b. Details of treatment equipment (please give details such as the number, type and capacity of each unit)

	No of units	Capacity of each unit
Incinerators:		
Plasma pyrolysis:		
Autoclaves:		
Microwave:		
Hydroclave:		
Shredder:		
Needle tip cutter or destroyer:		
Sharps encapsulation or concrete pit:		
Deep burial pits:		
Chemical disinfection:		
Any other treatment equipment:		

7. Contingency plan of common bio-medical waste treatment facility (CBWTF)(attach documents):

8. Details of directions or notices or legal actions if any during the period of earlier authorisation

9. Declaration:

   I do hereby declare that the statements made and information given above are true to the best of my knowledge and belief and that I have not concealed any information.

   I do also hereby undertake to provide any further information sought by the prescribed authority in relation to these rules and to fulfill any conditions stipulated by the prescribed authority.

Date ....   Signature of the applicant ....

Place ....   Designation of the applicant ....

FORM III
(See rule 10)
AUTHORISATION

(Authorisation for operating a facility for generation, collection, reception, treatment, storage, transport and disposal of biomedical wastes)

1. File number of authorisation and date of issue ....
2. M/s .... an occupier or operator of the facility located at .... is hereby granted an authorisation for;

   Activity   *Please tick*
   Generation, segregation
   Collection,
   Storage packaging
   Reception
   Transportation
   Treatment or processing or conversion
   Recycling
   Disposal or destruction
   use
   offering for sale, transfer
   Any other form of handling

3. M/s .... is hereby authorized for handling of biomedical waste as per the capacity given below;
   a. Number of beds of HCF:
   b. Number of healthcare facilities covered by CBMWTF: ....
   c. Installed treatment and disposal capacity: .... kg per day
   d. Area or distance covered by CBMWTF: ....
   e. Quantity of Biomedical waste handled, treated or disposed:
      Type of waste category   *Quantity permitted for handling*
      Yellow
      Red
      White (translucent)
      Blue

4. This authorisation shall be in force for a period of .... years from the date of issue.
5. This authorisation is subject to the conditions stated below and to such other conditions as may be specified in the rules for the time being in force under the Environment (Protection) Act, 1986.

Date ....   Signature ....

Place ....   Designation ....

Terms and conditions of authorisation *
1. The authorisation shall comply with the provisions of the Environment (Protection) Act, 1986 and the rules made thereunder.
2. The authorisation or its renewal shall be produced for inspection at the request of an officer authorised by the prescribed authority.
3. The person authorized shall not rent, lend, sell, transfer or otherwise transport the biomedical wastes without obtaining prior permission of the prescribed authority.
4. Any unauthorised change in personnel, equipment or working conditions as mentioned in the application by the person authorised shall constitute a breach of his authorisation.
5. It is the duty of the authorised person to take prior permission of the prescribed authority to close down the facility and such other terms and conditions may be stipulated by the prescribed authority.

FORM IV
(See rule 13)
ANNUAL REPORT

[To be submitted to the prescribed authority on or before 30th June every year for the period from January to December of the preceding year, by the occupier of health care facility (HCF) or common bio-medical waste treatment facility (CBWTF)]

Sl. No.	Particulars		
1.	Particulars of the occupier		
	a.	Name of the authorised person (occupier or operator of facility)	
	b.	Name of HCF or CBMWTF	:
	c.	Address for correspondence	:
	d.	Address of facility	
	e.	Tel. No., Fax. No.	:
	f.	E-mail ID	:
	g.	URL of Website	
	h.	GPS coordinates of HCF or CBMWTF	
	i.	Ownership of HCF or CBMWTF	: (State Government or Private or Semi Govt. or any other)
	j.	Status of authorisation under the Bio-Medical Waste (Management and Handling) Rules	: Authorisation No.: ……………………………………… valid up to ……………………………
	k.	Status of consents under Water Act and Air Act	: Valid up to:
2.	Type of healthcare facility		:
	a.	Bedded hospital	: No. of beds:
	b.	Non-bedded hospital (Clinic or Blood Bank or Clinical Laboratory or Research Institute or Veterinary Hospital or any other)	:
	c.	License number and its date of expiry	

3.	Details of CBMWTF:		
	a.	Number healthcare facilities covered by CBMWTF	:
	b.	No of beds covered by CBMWTF	:
	c.	Installed treatment and disposal capacity of CBMWTF:	: .... kg per day
	d.	Quantity of biomedical waste treated or disposed by CBMWTF	: .... kg/day
4.	Quantity of waste generated or disposed in kg per annum (on monthly average basis)		: Yellow category: .... Red category: .... White: .... Blue category: .... General solid waste: ....
5	Details of the storage, treatment, transportation, processing and disposal facility		
	a.	Details of the on-site storage facility	: Size:
			Capacity:
			Provision of on-site storage: (cold storage or any other provision)

b. Disposal facilities:

Type of treatment equipment	No. of units	Capacity Kg/day	Quantity treated or disposed in kg per annum
Incinerators:			
Plasma pyrolysis:			
Autoclaves:			
Microwave:			
Hydroclave:			
Shredder:			
Needle tip cutter or destroyer:			
Sharps encapsulation or concrete pit:			
Deep burial pits:			
Chemical disinfection:			
Any other treatment equipment:			

	c.	Quantity of recyclable wastes sold to authorized recyclers after treatment in kg per annum	: Red category (like plastic, glass etc.)
	d.	No of vehicles used for collection and transportation of biomedical waste	:
	e.	Details of incineration ash and ETP sludge generated and disposed during the treatment of wastes in kg per annum	Quantity generated / Where disposed Incineration Ash ETP sludge
	f.	Name of the common bio-medical waste treatment facility operator through which wastes are disposed of	:
	g.	List of member HCF not handed over bio-medical waste.	
6	Do you have bio-medical waste management committee? If yes, attach minutes of the meetings held during the reporting period		
7	Details trainings conducted on BMW		
	a.	Number of trainings conducted on BMW management.	
	b.	Number of personnel trained	
	c.	Number of personnel trained at the time of induction	
	d.	Number of personnel not undergone any training so far	
	e.	Whether standard manual for training is available?	
	f.	Any other information)	
8	Details of the accident occurred during the year		
	a.	Number of accidents occurred	
	b.	Number of the persons affected	

	c. Remedial action taken (please attach details if any)	
	d. Any fatality occurred, details.	
9.	Are you meeting the standards of air pollution from the incinerator? How many times in last year could not met the standards?	
	Details of continuous online emission monitoring systems installed	
10.	Liquid waste generated and treatment methods in place. How many times you have not met the standards in a year?	
11.	Is the disinfection method or sterilization meeting the log 4 standards? How many times you have not met the standards in a year?	
12.	Any other relevant information	: (Air Pollution Control Devices attached with the Incinerator)

Certified that the above report is for the period from
....
....
....
....

Name and Signature of the Head of the Institution

Date: ....
Place: ....

FORM V
(See rule 16)

Application for filing appeal against order passed by the prescribed **authority**

1. Name and address of the person applying for appeal :
2. Number, date of order and address of the authority which passed the order, against which appeal is being made (certified copy of order to be attached):
3. Ground on which the appeal is being made:
4. List of enclosures other than the order referred in para 2 against which appeal is being filed:

Signature ....

Date: ....   Name and Address..........................

Annexure G: Needle Stick Injury Report Form

Reporting of Needle Stick Injuries

Name and full address of hospital..

....

....

Needle stick sharp injury protocol:

Name of health care worker: ....

Category of heath care worker: ....

Employment no. ....

Date of needle stick/sharp injury ....

Date of reporting to casualty ....

Site and depth of injury ....

Nature of Injury: Needle Prick/Sharp Cut/Laceration/Splach of Fluids/Splattered Glass

Action taken in casualty: ....

Hep. B vaccination given:	Yes/No
HBIG:	Yes/No

If immunized: Date .... Intradermal/Intramuscular

Anti HBsAg Titre ....

HbsAg	Positive/Negative
HIV antibody	Postive/Negative

Information about source of contamination (if available)

- Whether the patient has symptoms of HIV infection or no symptoms
- Serum sent for: (Reports to be entered in follow up visit)
    01. Anti-HIV
    02. HBsAg
    03. Anti-HCV
    04. CD4/CD8 counts

Annexure H:
Incinarator Function Monitoring

Days	Time	Primary chamber		Secondary chamber temp (°C)	Surrounding of the incinerator
		Temp (°C)	Brick lining		
Monday					
Tuesday					
Wednesday					
Thursday					
Friday					
Saturday					
Sunday					

Signature

Name of Inspecting Officer

Note:
Comments on brick lining—Intact/Broken
Comments on surrounding of incinerator—Clean/Satisfactory/Dirty

Further Reading

1. Prussa A, Cirouit E and Rushbrook P. Safe Management of Waste from Health care Activities, WHO, 1999.
2. Park's. Textbook of Preventive and Social Medicine, 18th edition, Jabalpur, 2005.
3. Dhar GM, Rabbani I. Foundation of Community Medicine, Read Elsevier India Pvt Ltd, New Delhi, Ist edition, 2006.
4. Sharma, Maduri. Hosptial waste management and its monitoring, Jaypee Brothers Medical Publishers (P) Ltd, New Delhi, 2002.
5. Faisal Khan Mohd. Hospital waste management, principles and guidelines, Kanishka Publishers, New Delhi, 2004.
6. Manual for control of hospital associated infections (SOP), NACO, MOHFW, GOI,1999.
7. Cedric B, Sharma DK, Goyal RC. A practical guide to hospital planning and management,Voluntary Health Association of India, New Delhi, 1999.
8. World Alliance for Patient Safety, Forward Programme WHO, 2005.
9. IGNOU. Certificate in Health care Waste Management, BHM 002, SHOS, IGNOU, New Delhi.
10. Govt of India. Biomedical Waste (Management and Handling) Rules, 1998, The Gazette of India. Ministry of Environment and Forest, New Delhi, 20th July, 1998.
11. Manual on hospital waste management, CPCB, Ministry of Environment and Forest, 2001.
12. Related Websites:
    www.who.int/patientsafety
    www.no-harm.org
    www.toxiclink.org
    www.healthcarewaste.org
    http//cpcb.envfor.nic.in/cpcb
    www.cpcb.nic.in
13. Biomedical Waste Management Rules 2016.